Principles and Practices of Relational Psychotherapy

This book provides an overview of the basic principles in relational therapy, which, in combination with the latest research about the significance of the therapeutic relationship, makes it possible to present practical therapeutic tools and techniques to help the therapist make optimal use of the interaction between patient and therapist.

It presents models and concepts in relational psychotherapy that may contribute to the patient's development of relational and emotional competence, and to more authentic and meaningful ways of living with oneself and others. The book specially emphasizes the significance of the mutually constructed emotional interplay as the material for key experiences in the development of the patient – and therapist.

The focus is on the usefulness of relational principles and research findings in psychotherapies of shorter duration, in primary care, psychiatric clinics, and private practice.

Rich in clinical examples, *Principles and Practices of Relational Psychotherapy* is an extremely useful resource for psychotherapists and clinical psychologists in training and practice.

Rolf Holmqvist is a Professor of Clinical Psychology at Linköping University, Sweden, where he researches and teaches in psychotherapy. He has worked as a psychotherapist and clinical supervisor for 50 years.

Principles and Practices of Relational Psychotherapy

Rolf Holmqvist

Routledge
Taylor & Francis Group

LONDON AND NEW YORK

Cover image: © Getty Images

First published 2022
by Routledge
4 Park Square, Milton Park, Abingdon, Oxon OX14 4RN

and by Routledge
605 Third Avenue, New York, NY 10158

Routledge is an imprint of the Taylor & Francis Group, an informa business

© 2022 Rolf Holmqvist

British Library Cataloguing-in-Publication Data
A catalogue record for this book is available from the British Library

Library of Congress Cataloging-in-Publication Data
Names: Holmqvist, Rolf, 1948- author.
Title: Principles and practices of relational psychotherapy / Rolf Holmqvist.
Description: Milton Park, Abingdon, Oxon ; New York, NY : Routledge, 2022. | Includes bibliographical references and index.
Identifiers: LCCN 2021037074 (print) | LCCN 2021037075 (ebook) | ISBN 9780367461010 (hardback) | ISBN 9780367461027 (paperback) | ISBN 9781003026914 (ebook)
Subjects: LCSH: Interpersonal psychotherapy. | Psychotherapist and patient.
Classification: LCC RC489.I55 H65 2022 (print) | LCC RC489.I55 (ebook) | DDC 616.89/14--dc23
LC record available at https://lccn.loc.gov/2021037074
LC ebook record available at https://lccn.loc.gov/2021037075

ISBN: 978-0-367-46101-0 (hbk)
ISBN: 978-0-367-46102-7 (pbk)
ISBN: 978-1-003-02691-4 (ebk)

DOI: 10.4324/9781003026914

Typeset in Times
by MPS Limited, Dehradun

Contents

Foreword

A basic dimension in human life straddles separateness and relatedness. Not many years ago, psychotherapy students were taught that life starts in an autistic phase, in primary narcissism. Now, we know that newborn children relate from their first hour (Luyten, Mayes, Target, & Fonagy, 2012; Meltzoff & Moore, 1998; Tronick, 2007). Capacity to be alone and ability to relate, relishing independence and self-reliance versus enjoying dependence and trustfulness, are states of the mind that grow in interaction from the beginning. Alone in the forest, a person may feel the vital mental presence of others. And in the most intimate or socially engaging context, a person may feel intensely lonely.

In the current psychotherapy world, there is a move towards the autonomy pole. Many therapy methods promote the idea that the suffering person should take charge of his or her life, challenge himself or herself, and practise mentally. Exposure treatment, mindfulness meditation, and affect regulation strategies are practised by the person himself or herself, albeit sometimes supported by a therapist-coach. As Safran (2016) noted, mindfulness meditation in Eastern traditions has been used both to increase the individual's "self-power" and to endorse "other-power", that is, surrender to trust in an inspiring person. In Western psychotherapy, the use of mindfulness for self-power is predominant.

One reason for the focus on autonomy in contemporary psychotherapy is certainly the general Western ideal of the self-reliant person (Cushman, 1996). "Institutionalized individualistic", modern people strive to leave behind ties to social class, ethnicity, religion, and kinship (Beck & Beck-Gernsheim, 2002). A goal for human development is to become flexible, also in human relationships, implying widened life possibilities – and precariousness for the socially vulnerable (Layton, 2014).

Techniques for individuals may certainly be effective and often have substantial research evidence. It is, however, suggestive that contemporary psychotherapy research strongly supports the significance of the therapeutic relationship for successful outcome. Innumerable studies show that the quality of the relationship between patient and therapist has at least as much importance for the effects of therapy as the specific technique (Wampold & Imel, 2015).

Psychoanalytic therapies have for decades emphasized the importance of observing and reflecting on the therapeutic relationship. Until recently, the model was that the expert-therapist interpreted the historical meanings of the patient's relating patterns, particularly in the interaction with the therapist. This perspective is fundamentally individualistic; the expert applies his or her technique in order to uncover the meaning of how the other relates to him or her.

Practice and research

Psychoanalytic authors, beginning with Freud, have considered their theories to be scientifically based (Brenner, 1968; Waelder, 1962). They have, however, often shunned meddling with empirical psychotherapy research. Despite strong empirical evidence for relational interventions, psychoanalytic authors, albeit with many noteworthy exceptions, have not, for instance, shown interest in systematic studies of the transference-countertransference interaction, a basic concept in psychoanalytic practice. This is even more so among relational psychoanalytic authors (Hoffman, 2009a).

Relational theorists often insist that the mutual interplay in the therapeutic relationship is too subtle to measure or categorize with scientific tools (Hoffman, 2009a; Stern, 2013a). There is truth in this. To study the interaction in psychotherapy in depth is complicated. Strupp, a doyen in the field of psychotherapy research, wrote: "Given the uniqueness of every therapeutic dyad and the multitude of relevant interacting variables influencing the course of treatment, the 'empirical validation' of any therapy is utterly illusory" (Strupp, 2001, p. 613).

But even so, avoidance of potentially valuable knowledge from empirical science is unhealthy and favours sectarianism. In our days of information bubbles, it is important to listen to diverse knowledge sources, to meet "the hard questions" (Luyten, 2015; Spence, 1994). A dialogue between findings and concepts in relational therapy and empirical studies of the therapeutic relationship may advance knowledge and creativity in both areas.

This book is written from the outside. The author is not a psychoanalyst. The motive for writing the book is to understand how knowledge from relational psychoanalysis can be combined with empirical findings in order to further outcome in different treatment contexts. Principles in relational therapy are discussed in the light of findings from empirical studies and used in illustrations of situations in routine therapy work in clinics and primary care services where conventional psychoanalytic methods would neither be feasible nor appropriate. Arguably, the vast majority of real-life psychodynamic and relational treatments, particularly if they are publicly financed, are shorter and with lower session frequency than therapies usually described in the psychoanalytic relational literature. The purpose of the book is to reflect on the possibilities, difficulties, and limitations of using relational understanding in such treatments.

In order to simplify the reading, patients are in general male and therapists are female. No distinctions will be made between the concepts psychoanalytic and psychodynamic except where differences between them are discussed. The concept relational will be used in a broad sense, encompassing both ideas from relational psychoanalysts, from other schools defining themselves as relational and from researchers who use a relational perspective.

Part I
Principles

1   Invitation

This book takes its starting point in two traditions: the psychoanalytic re-lational movement and empirical psychotherapy studies. Some persons would consider this an oxymoronic project. The spirits and sensibilities in these theoretical traditions may seem incompatible (Hoffman, 2009a; Lingiardi, Holmqvist, & Safran, 2016). Nonetheless, they both, to a large extent, focus on the therapeutic relationship and how to use it for the im-provement and growth of the patient. The knowledge basis in relational therapy is the large number of case studies that describe and reflect on subtleties in the interplay between patient and therapist. Empirical research also focuses on the relationship, but with other methodological tools. Some of them are, to be sure, blunt for subtle observations. But the range of different degrees of fineness in methods should impress even sceptics.

Focus on the therapeutic interplay

Relational therapy uses curiosity on the affective aspects of the therapeutic relationship to achieve its effects. The human ability to actively reflect on the motives and reasons for her own and others' behaviour in interaction is basic to a constructive and self-fulfilling life. Problems in psychological and relational functioning can be characterized as inhibitions and limitations of this reflecting ability (Fonagy, Luyten, & Allison, 2015).

The human species, homo sapiens, stands out among primates by the size of its neocortex (Kanai et al., 2012; Kochiyama et al., 2018). The size of the neocortex is associated with the capacity to interact in social networks. The Neanderthals had larger visual cortex but smaller neocortex. They needed their sight but could not compete with homo sapiens' ability to reflect on complex interactions. The meaning of our subspecies name, *homo sapiens sapiens,* can be understood to mean the "human who knows that she knows". She can reflect on her own cognitive and relational experiences (Hare & Woods, 2020).

A great potential in human interaction is the ability to talk about others, to gossip, to communicate knowledge about the network. The capacity to build security in relationships and to be curious about the dynamics of social

DOI: 10.4324/9781003026914-1

relating is the basis for human life – and for human trouble. This curiosity starts at the beginning of life, stimulated in the primary relationships. Good caregivers encourage the child to attend to affects, to find meaning in relationships, and to ask about the ongoing relationship and about social experiences with others (Allison & Fonagy, 2016; Tronick, 1998).

Freud's curiosity

One of the foundational works of psychoanalysis is Freud's case description *Bruchstücke einer Hysterie-Analyse* ("Fragments of an Analysis of a Case of Hysteria"; Freud, 1905). In this paper, Freud tried to figure out why his patient Dora abruptly left their therapy. Freud could have left the matter with excuses about the patient's lack of motivation or young age. Instead, he grappled with ideas about what had happened between them, what conscious and unconscious thoughts and feelings their relationship had activated. He did what humans are wired to do, he tried to understand the interaction between them.

This was one of the first times Freud used the concept transference, meaning the patient's transferring previously experienced relational patterns to a new relationship. It was a large step forward in the science of psychotherapy; a new way to understand problematic emotional reactions was opened. However, what Freud did not analyze was the complexities in his own reactions to Dora. There, his curiosity stopped. Decade-long theoretical and clinical thinking has rectified him on this point (Mahoney, 1996, 2005). Curiosity on the countertransference and on the therapeutic interaction has led to Relational psychotherapy.

Relationships are conflictual

Human relational development, as a child or as a patient, does not come off linearly. On the contrary, relationships are fraught with hassles, conflicts, misunderstandings, reparative attempts, and new failures (Bazzano, 2014; Sidnell, 2016; Tronick, 1998). Humans enter relationships with different expectations, different representational perspectives, different value systems, incongruent affects, colliding wishes, and intentions (Pizer, 1998; Slavin & Kriegman, 1998). Our longing to be recognized and understood is continuously thwarted, in fact or in fantasy (Benjamin, 1988). Conflicts are the energy of relational development. Relational therapy is Hegelian in considering conflicts as constructive and creative.

The visible therapist

A primary principle in relational therapy is to focus on the therapeutic relationship as material for understanding and vehicle for change. It is an important task for the therapist to contribute to the creation of a vital relationship with the patient. A person cannot relate to another person who does not relate. The patient needs a therapist who relates as much as the therapist needs a patient who relates. Or who plays, to use Winnicott's (1971a, p. 54) felicitous word.

The challenge in relational therapy is to be fully in the relationship and at the same time to reflect on it; to be "mindful in action" (Safran & Muran, 2000). The therapist is present and participating while at the same time observing the interaction (Sullivan, 1940). Relational sensibility, the ability to be aware of and sensitively communicate about intricate fluctuations in the therapeutic interplay, is the therapist's most important tool. Other techniques and methods are optional within a large range.

Uniqueness

Social systems have their unique characteristics, partly determined by preceding factors and partly by the interaction that emerges. Tolstoy's introductory comment in Anna Karenina that each unhappy family is unhappy in its own way, but all happy families are similar is brilliant but not true. Happy families are happy in their own ways, too.

In relational therapy, the uniqueness is "consequential" in the sense that it has bearing on the treatment, in contrast to unique cases of somatic illnesses like diabetes or ulcerative colitis. For somatic states, the physician's technical expertise is necessary and usually sufficient. As long as the physician understands the physiological conditions, the contact with the patient as a person is of less importance. She can, in principle, be replaced as long as the expertise on the illness is retained. This perspective is also predominant in psychotherapy methods that focus on treatment of limited problems and syndromes rather than on the patient as a person. In relational treatment, however, the therapist is not replaceable. The interaction with the unique therapist is part of the material that the therapy focuses on.

Relational complexity

Theorists and researchers from various theoretical vantage points have pointed to the need to use complex models for understanding change processes in psychotherapy (Gelo & Salvatore, 2016). Change is often nonlinear, sudden, and discontinuous (Hayes, Laurenceau, & Cardaciotto, 2008). Although psychotherapy has been described as "ultimate low in technology" (Wampold & Imel, 2015), it is also one of the most complex professional activities that exist. Each interactional step requires immediate decisions based on complicated and often subtle signals coming from the patient's and the therapist's trait-based patterns and current emotional state. Dynamic non-linear models have been suggested as theoretical and empirical tools by relational therapists and empirical researchers (Atzil-Slonim & Tschacher, 2020; Seligman, 2005). The concepts non-linear and dynamic imply that the therapeutic process is open and unpredictable. The trait characteristics of the participants do not determine the system's transformations, it has emergent and recursive qualities. Previous interpersonal experiences may leave tracks in the mind as common pathways or interactional templates (Freud, 1912a, 1912b) but their usefulness for predicting the system's properties and alterations is limited.

Stiles, Honos-Webb, and Surko (1998) gave a metaphorical description of the difficulty to predict psychotherapy processes when they compared therapeutic interaction with ballistics, the science about artillery, about trajectories of bullets and rockets. Psychotherapy is not like the firing of a cannonball. To predict the movement of a projectile through the air, the laws of classical mechanics suffice: knowledge about cannon pipe, projectile, wind, air pressure, and moisture. To predict the movement in therapy is impossible. The large number of factors that interact in complicated patterns continuously change the course of the therapeutic dialogue. The mutual interaction entails ever shifting feelings and fantasies, unexpected formulations, and reactions. If the therapist would follow a manual mechanically, the therapy would become meaningless. "what has happened can be narrated, but what is happening cannot be narrated" (Tronick, 2003, p. 477).

Affective interplay

In relational therapy, the affective interplay between patient and therapist is in focus. Affects have basic significance as change agents (Aafjes-van Doorn & Barber, 2017; Greenberg & Pascual-Leone, 2006). Affects are what make relationships vital and meaningful. Thoughtful reflection is a guide in social situations but affects give them life. In many therapy methods, the therapist focuses on the patient's feelings. In relational therapy, the therapist asks herself what she feels at the same time as she explores the emotional interaction with the patient.

Two-person perspective

The focus on the mutual affective interaction in relational therapy points to its major defining characteristic: the two-person perspective. Therapy interaction is co-constructed, both participants contribute continuously to the process. This means that the idea of exploring recurrent relational patterns becomes problematic. If material brought by the patient like memories, fantasies, fears, expectations, emotions, is continuously and inexorably remoulded in the shared dialog, mutually understood, co-created, the question of roots in the patient's previous experiences becomes less meaningful. The therapy is an ongoing dialectic between using recurrent interactional patterns and creating new ways of being together.

Psychoanalysis and psychotherapy

Almost since its inception, psychoanalysts have discussed if the principles in Freud's psychoanalytic theories and techniques can be used in other treatment formats and modalities. In 1919, Freud argued that the press for shorter treatments "will compel us to alloy the pure gold of analysis ... with the copper of suggestion" (pp. 167–168). Freud's view of a contrast between exploration and suggestion has in our days been superseded by other opposites. One is between longer, open-ended treatments with personal growth as goal versus more active psychodynamic methods with circumscribed, sometimes symptom-focused, objectives. Another is between therapies based on the medical model of therapist-treating-patient and relational two-person models.

Although many authors have argued for a distinction between psychoanalysis and therapies that do not go to the infantile roots of the patient's experiences, using the couch and therapist neutrality as tools (Gill, 1954; Glover, 1954), Freud already in 1914 argued that any therapy that takes as starting points transference and resistance could be called psychoanalysis. During the past half-century, psychoanalytic theorists have by and large accepted that treatments that diverge from psychoanalytic techniques in their classical form may be valuable ways of working with psychoanalytical principles. A notable example is Gill, for many years, a leading proponent of an orthodox view of psychoanalysis and later one of the forerunners of relational therapy. In a paper (1984), he explicitly rejected his former position and questioned the mandatory use of the couch and several weekly sessions.

Modern definitions of psychoanalytic treatment focus on the therapeutic approach rather than on extrinsic criteria. A common idea is that the principle for analytically based therapies should be the therapist's *intention* (Cooper, 2010; Mitchell, 2000; Tublin, 2018). If the intention is to elicit and inspire the patient's curiosity on his mental world, it is psychoanalysis.

Time-limited and targeted psychodynamic therapies

"Pluralism is the hallmark of 21st century psychoanalytic discourse" (Gabbard, 2007, p. 559). Time-limited and goal-focused psychoanalytic therapies have proliferated in the past half-century (Bateman & Fonagy, 2006; Luborsky, 1984; Malan, 1963; Mann, 1973; Sifneos,1979; Yeomans, Clarkin, & Kernberg, 2014). To different degrees, these therapies focus on specific themes or problems, such as circumscribed interpersonal conflicts, diagnosis categories, or problems with specific psychological competencies.

A manualized method for working with the patient's relationship themes as they emerge between therapist and patient is Supportive-Expressive (SE) therapy (Luborsky, 1984; Luborsky & Crits-Christoph, 1990). This method uses a standardized method for identifying relationship patterns, the Core Conflictual Relationship Themes (CCRT). In contrast to relational therapy, an explicit ambition in SE therapy is to find recurrent patterns in the patient's interaction, making "accurate" interpretations possible.

Several affect-focused therapies are also based on psychodynamic principles. Intensive Short-Term Dynamic Therapy (ISTDP; Davanloo, 1995), Affect-Phobia Therapy (APT, McCullough et al., 2003), and Accelerated Experiential Dynamic Psychotherapy (AEDP; Fosha, 2000) are examples of therapies that use psychodynamic principles in targeted and systematic ways. These therapies use more active and expressive techniques than the classical psychoanalytic listening and interpretative stance, but they are based on aspects of psychoanalytic theory: resistance, repressed intentions, and fantasies, and on the transference model (Malan, 1963).

In contrast to these therapies with brand names, relational psychoanalysis and relational therapy have grown in a more organic and gradual way out of psychoanalysis. The demarcation between traditional psychoanalysis and relational psychotherapy is in no way strict; relational perspectives are common in main-stream psychoanalysis (Fonagy & Campbell, 2015). In contrast to the affect-focused therapies, relational treatment comes in both psychoanalytic and psychotherapeutic treatment formats without any clear distinction.

Relational psychotherapy shuns treatment manuals and guidelines. Brief Relational Therapy (BRT; Safran & Muran, 2000) is an example of a time-limited relational therapy. Although it is marketed as a "treatment guide", it has few of the characteristics of manuals. In contrast to other time-limited dynamic therapies, the patient and therapist are not recommended to focus on and stick to a specific theme or problem area (Safran, 2002). Instead, the mutual work between patient and therapist on the problems that the patient presents is allowed to evolve during the treatment, using urgency, meaningfulness, and emotional charge as guides in the developing therapy.

Time-limited and endless

Freud's last paper was entitled *Die endliche und die unendliche Analyse* ("Analysis terminable and interminable", (1937). One reason for him to write this article was the fact that psychoanalytic treatments had become successively longer over the years. In view of contemporary trends away from year-long psychoanalytic therapies to shorter treatments, often with circumscribed goals, it is of interest to reflect on the meaning of time in psychotherapy.

There is to be sure a practical side to this issue; persons have limited time and money, and there is no more reason to spend years in a therapist's office than to go to the dentist continuously. People come to therapists because they have problems in life, and they want the problems to be addressed in order to make life more worth living.

In professional relations with a physician or a craftsman, time is due to the solution of the problem. Professional contacts with coaches and mentors also have time limits, although usually vaguer. The mentor is a dedicated person who follows the client during a stretch of life as long as the relationship is creative, meaningful, productive. In relationships with friends and family, in contrast, there is obviously no apparent task to accomplish. Friends are not primarily for problem solving; one of the points of having a friendship is that it has no time limit.

So, what is a therapist? Sometimes like a craftsman when a circumscribed problem can be identified and solved. Sometimes, somewhat of a friend. But the most useful metaphor for a therapist may be a mentor. A person who engages in the patient's life for specific purposes. Many psychotherapists these days probably consider themselves to be on the border between mentor and craftsman, with clear goals and time limits. Relational therapists, in contrast, feel more at home on the border between mentor and friend (BCPSG, 2018a, 2018b).

Discovery, creation, and time limits

If the goal in treatment is to uncover dysfunctional relational patterns, according to the "Sherlock Holmes" model (Spence, 1982, 1987), treatment time can be limited. Although the process may be long, in the end, the patient has become aware of the significant aspects of his repressed dispositions. Clichés like "fully analyzed" and "remaining blind spots" belong to this model of therapy.

In relational therapy, the contextualization of retrieved experiences in the ongoing interaction implies a mutual search for new meanings in relationships, for construal of a potential space of unmet possibilities. "The task is not to tease apart the elements [that] belong to each individual participating in it; ... the analytic task involves an attempt to describe as fully as possible the specific nature of the experience of the interplay of individual subjectivity and inter-subjectivity" (Ogden, 1994a, p. 4). Important life experiences are grain for the creative intersubjective mill rather than events to be uncovered (Stern, 1983, 1997). When the therapy model moves to a greater emphasis on the emergence of heretofore unformulated, mutually created, emergent experiences in the therapeutic relationship, the conception of time in therapy changes. New experiences are always possible to make. The limit to the creative ability of the therapeutic couple is their curiousness and energy. Therapy can last as long as the participants find it meaningful. It is like the artist who works on the same theme for many years, creating ever new and meaningful expressions.

Growth in psychotherapy

A child grows in its own pace, as does friendship. Is it possible to achieve emotional growth in a limited number of sessions? The response would seem to be obvious: growth needs time. Another response could be that it is a matter of intensity; a deep and emotionally moving shared experience may imply immediate emotional growth in the patient – and therapist (Mearns & Cooper, 2005; Stern, 2004a).

The therapist-intervention → patient-reaction model is basic to most psychological treatments, including psychoanalytic therapies. The therapist makes an intervention, such as an interpretation and awaits the patient's response. Such treatment models rely on the idea that there are specific techniques that potentially produce specific change.

In contrast, therapies like relational therapy and humanistic therapies are based on the idea that humans develop in relationships, that the relationship is the prime intervention although the therapist may use a specific stance or a way of responding to the patient that follows a specific model. In order to make the idea comprehensible, an everyday illustration may help:

The boy is scared of darkness. His mother considers using various tricks and steps to help her boy, like gradually exposing him to dark places. Solution-oriented interventions like these are made in a relational context: the mother negotiates with her boy, tries to figure out what would be possible to suggest, what the boy would refuse to do. The boy, perhaps distraught by fear of what his mother might suggest, tries to understand when it is possible to say no and when he has to accept the mother's ideas, all in the context of their mutual relationship.

Imagine that the mother suggests that the boy should go into a dark room. The boy accepts somewhat hesitatingly. When she tries to close the door in order to make it really dark, he becomes frightened and runs out. The mother soothes the crying boy. The boy tries again but comes out even faster. After a few attempts, the mother becomes impatient and tries to persuade the boy to stay a few more seconds. The emotional tension between them will increase.

In this process, the mother and the boy find their own ways of handling fear, hope, disappointment, impatience, and joy. They may argue, be angry at each other, become friends again, and enjoy their cooperation. They will find their own rhythm of emotional interaction, with ruptures and repairs (Tronick, 1998). Perhaps they create a play situation, perhaps they have to deal with a lock in their relating. Although ways of negotiating conflicts are not transferable among different situations (Tronick, 2003), the basic feeling that "I am able to handle complicated relational situations" grows in the boy.

The goal is to help the boy overcome his fear of darkness, but the effect of the negotiations and the more or less successful activities is not only, and not primarily, that the boy learns to manage his fears. The main effect is that both move along a little bit in their understanding of relational complexities. This does not mean that the "techniques" they use are irrelevant. The systematic exposure to darkness that the mother suggests is probably helpful. The challenges in their mutual attempts are necessary for the relational growth to proceed. The unformulated "goal" is that the boy grows as an agentic and mentalizing young person, although this is not at all the intention of the mother. The interaction is based on, and influences, their ways of being together, their confidence in each, how ruptures are handled, their images of how they may deal with complicated situations in the future. The interaction is engaged and goal-directed, they are significant persons, "charged others", to each other (BCPSG, 2018a, 2018b). The growth process has no time limit; the participants will know when it is time to stop.

What is enough, when is it time to stop?

The discussion so far has suggested that there are different perspectives on the duration of change processes in therapy. It may be helpful to summarize them.

The Kairos perspective

Change may be momentary. Although therapeutic presence probably increases the probability for change to take place, decisive experiences may be sudden and unplanned (Duarte et al., 2020; Fosshage, 2003). Stern et al. (1998, 2004a, 2004b) described how therapy may "move along" until it reaches a "present moment", characterized by intensified affect, which can develop to a "now moment" when the intersubjective feelings between patient and therapist come in focus, and often get strained. If attended to, such occasions may become a "moment of meeting", a Kairos moment, sometimes implying that a new relational structure between therapist and patient emerges (Lord, 2017; Mearns & Cooper, 2005). These moments of meeting with mutual experiences of heightened affectivity may result in new states of intersubjectivity that may configure the patient's procedural knowledge of being with others in new ways (BCPSG, 2010).

Building relational skills

One aim of relational therapy is to improve the patient's relational skills: to improve mentalizing, to increase the ability to observe the mind's workings, to become aware of disavowed affects. Such goals can be defined, progress evaluated. For shorter treatments aimed at symptom reduction, several studies have shown that patients develop at their own pace; in some therapies, symptom reduction is steep, other therapies need more time (Falkenström et al., 2016; Reese, Toland, & Hopkins, 2011). There are no studies on such "good-enough" models for longer treatments with relational goals, but it is reasonable to assume that similar models are applicable; circumscribed goals need less time, but therapies develop in their own pace.

Authentic relating

A wider purpose of relational therapy is to help persons develop their capacity to live more genuinely, meaningfully, and worthy, to appreciate relationships, to make symptoms and problems understandable in a life perspective. Such development may come from a row of Kairos moments or from slowly growing understanding that relationships can be experienced in new ways. These are radical, sea-changing, seminal developments that sometimes turn the patient's life upside down. They take the time it takes.

Spirit and techniques in relational therapy

The relational psychotherapeutic movement is relational. The most reasonable "father" of relational therapy, Stephen Mitchell, was strongly opposed to the idea of any kind of canonical textbook about relational therapy (Davies, 2018) and to seeing himself as the founder. The relational tradition has been created by many persons in a continuously evolving exchange of ideas and perspectives. Although there are principles and leading thoughts, no one would assume responsibility to decide on the boundaries of relational thought (Bass, 2014; Davies, 2018).

The openness and multiplicity in the relational movement may imply a risk that relational therapy becomes contourless – and perhaps cautious (Davies, 2018; Tublin, 2018). Interestingly, and paradoxically, despite the openness among relational authors to experiment with psychoanalytic principles, and the openness to influence from contemporary ideas about social issues, there is a striking lack of curiosity about fertilizing combinations between relational therapy and other psychotherapy methods, notably cognitive behavioural therapies (Wachtel, 2018). Recent attempts to question tenets in relational theory emphasize the connection with older psychoanalytic concepts rather than to traditions outside psychoanalysis (Aron, Grand, & Slochower, 2018a, 2018b). The "psychoanalytic third" (Aron, 1999), the intellectual and clinical community of psychoanalytic journals, conferences, and networks, seems to frame and limit curiosity.

The spirit

The basic spirit of relational therapy is spontaneity in the therapeutic relationship, openness to the emergence of feelings, recollections, fantasies, strivings, despair, and hope in the therapeutic dyad (Hoffman, 1998). The idea of *emergence* is at the heart. Although the patient brings narratives and reflections to the session, the main therapeutic material is what emerges in the interaction. The spirit is to let the unknown happen rather than to discover what was once there.

Expertise

Skilful performance can often be described as tacit knowledge, as "the observance of a set of rules which are not known as such to the person following them" (Polanyi, 1958, p. 49). Professional competence is often procedural rather than declarative and often transferred by modelling, like old ways of learning a craft from expert masters.

In psychoanalysis, two ways of mediating competence have been dominating. One is to rely on standard method texts (Etchegoyen, 1991; Freud, 1911, 1912a, 1912b,; 1913, 1914 Greenson, 1967); the other is personal therapy and supervision. Both ways fall back on tradition and authority-based knowledge rather than on scientific discoveries or the student's curiosity and creativity. Such learning methods may be excellent if properly handled. But they may also lead to conservatism – and rebellion. Relational therapists often see themselves as rebels. A slogan has been to "throw away the book" (Hoffman, 1996). Standard ingredients of psychoanalytic technique have been subject to debate and rejection.

But rebelliousness needs defenders of old mores. It is uncertain to what extent defenders are available. "Issues that had been controversial a decade ago in psychoanalytic psychotherapy are mostly no longer so. There is, for example, little discussion now about the advantages or disadvantages of a relational approach: The overwhelming evidence favoring an interpersonal frame of reference for both development and adult functioning is generally accepted" (Fonagy, Allison & Campbell, 2019). And Mayes et al. (2015): "the language of psychodynamic thought has become more relational and experience-near" (p. 529).

Relational theory in a broad sense has become mainstream.

Deliberate technique and implicit relating

Whereas the theoretical development in relational therapy has been thorough and pervasive, the progress in therapeutic approach and method is basically left to personal initiatives. A leading idea is that implicit aspects of therapeutic relating are important for constructive results. The scale between implicit and explicit has many points. Interactional exchange may be completely out of awareness, it may be implicit but possible to capture with close attention, it may be apparent but out of focus, it may be deliberate, with many points in between.

Relational therapy focuses on these nuances. The therapist is supposed to attend to subtle emotional exchanges, sometimes hardly detectable. Bach (2006) admonishes the therapist to "pay very close attention in a particular kind of way" (p. 132) and Bass (2014) encourages the therapist "to listen carefully, with dedicated, highly concentrated attention to their patient's experience" (p. 668).

Engagement in the therapeutic relationship

Treatments are usually defined by techniques and methods. Relational therapy is easier identified by ideas, by its spirit. Few techniques would be proscribed (Tublin, 2011, 2018). Giving homework is not a commonly used tool in relational therapy, but the relational consequences of a homework assignment may be quite useful to work with.

Engagement is hard to define. Think of a band playing jazz: they may find melody, rhythm, harmonics but what makes the music is that they are dedicated, curious on divergencies, and playful. Knoblauch (2018), referring to Bucci (1997), calls such interaction subsymbolic. The interaction in the therapeutic dyad can be likened with the balance between synchronicity and asynchronicity (Knoblauch, 2018, p. 155).

Cure, knowledge, and truth

Psychoanalysis has a history of ambivalence towards quick and easy results. On several occasions, Freud denounced the value of psychoanalysis as symptom treatment. Especially, he warned about short and successful treatments that gave therapists increased self-esteem but did not contribute to knowledge (Freud, 1918, 1933). However, most persons do not enter therapy to further their knowledge. They want to understand and learn how to grapple with challenges in their ways of living. Although alleviation of discrete symptoms is not often a reason for a person who purposefully looks for a relational therapist, he certainly wants to come to grips with his relational and existential problems. Can a therapist content herself with saying that the patient knows more about his depression although it was not improved?

In a world where quick, straightforward, and often superficial solutions for mental problems are sought for, it is a challenge to argue for therapies with aims such as enhanced feelings of vitality and meaningfulness.

Relational therapy is sometimes criticized for focusing on the immediate interaction, jeopardizing interest in the patient's unconscious world, in his "private madness" (Green, 1986, 1995). Bolognini (1997), for instance, warned for empathism instead of empathy, meaning superficial niceness instead of true understanding. Kernberg (2001, p. 542) described the risk of "intersubjectivity as a seduction into a superficial interpersonal relationship [leading to] ... unconscious acting out of countertransference as a major consequence".

The age-old trauma issue has become symbolic in this discussion. Should traumatic experiences as such be targeted or rather the patient's fantasy elaborations around such experiences, the mental structures and the patient's agency? Busch (2010) argued that there is an obsession with the patient as a victim in some schools, therapy may inadvertently transform the subject to a victim of relational traumas rather than as the creator and owner of his mind. "Psychoanalysis has become about comfort, soothing and safety ... while passion, danger and desire have disappeared" (p. 91).

This is obviously a simplification. There is no contradiction between confirming the patient's experience of himself as a victim of traumatic experiences and an ambition to understand the subjective agency in the situations and their aftermath (Slavin & Pollock, 1997). It may be true that a spontaneous, active dialogue might stimulate to more care and concern about the patient, whereas a more reticent approach can make space for other reactions. But neutrality does not prevent mutual enactments or bastions (Baranger, Baranger, & Mom, 1983). Whether silent or talkative, the therapist's task is to find new ways for the patient to live with the trauma (Davies & Frawley, 1992).

Psychotherapeutic means and goals

Psychotherapy is a health care activity. The aim is to improve the patient's functioning, in relation to himself or others. Patients may want to attain an array of different goals, not always clear at the outset. But basically, mental health is always the raison d'être of psychotherapy. Without an effort to ameliorate mental suffering, psychotherapy becomes intellectual pastime or conversations about the hardships of life.

Some researchers have argued for a distinction between psychological treatment and psychotherapy (Barlow, 2004). Psychological treatments are based on scientifically tested techniques aimed at specified and circum-scribed symptoms and problems, whereas psychotherapy, according to Barlow, is more broadly focused on relational problems without clear links between intervention and goal.

This argument has reason in the sense that some interventions do in fact influence behaviours in specific ways. However, the only technique with an experimentally shown link between intervention and problem reduction is exposure for anxiety. The scientistic idea of circumscribed symptoms or problems that can be cured by specific techniques is inadequate for most patient situations. It is based on an inappropriate comparison with somatic problems. A broken knee can be cured with one method, pneumonia with another, although both problems are in the same patient. But a person with depression and aggressive impulsivity must be treated as the person he is, with a view of the patient as a person expressing his problems in different ways.

Based on this view of psychological problems, relational therapy is *person-centred* rather than problem- or disorder-centred (Glas, 2019; Luyten et al., 2012). The idea of symptom substitution, meaning that symptoms change expression if the basic conflict is not uncovered, is mechanical, but the gist of it, that problems can be expressed in different ways during life, is still valid. Longitudinal studies on psychiatric patients indicate that symptoms may change over time; what is constant is the tendency to get emotional problems (Caspi & Moffitt, 2018).

Symptom and meaning: an illustration

The relational stance is engagement with the patient rather than a planned treatment approach. "In an engaged relationship, a process of moving through the other is set in motion that catalyzes the emergence of more complex and fluid human capacities for relationship" (BCPSG, 2018b, p. 303). An illustration:

The patient, Arthur, comes to his primary care service with recurrent headaches, tiredness, lack of appetite and energy, sleeping difficulties, and anxiety bouts in the mornings. Several psychiatric diagnoses seem possible. His general practitioner (GP) refers him to a psychotherapist.

The problems started several years ago when Arthur and his wife got a child that they feared would be handicapped. Although things went all right with the baby, Arthur became cheerless and gloomy, and he also started to get anxiety bouts in the morning. His wife tried to talk with him about it, but he became silent and went by himself. From time to time, he has stayed home from work, and finally his employer told him that he must get help.

The therapist gets the impression that he is a serious and melancholic man. She asks him about details in his life to get a picture of who he is. Particularly, she tries to figure out what the fear of getting a handicapped child may have meant to him. When she asks, he is clearly reluctant to enlarge on it. She comments on that. He seems to get irritated, and she feels that she should perhaps be careful when asking about history. Instead, she tries to direct his attention to his current situation. After some discussion, he accepts to monitor and write down his feelings and thoughts in the mornings, as this seems to be the time of the day when things are worst for him. When he comes back after a week, he has no notes. He says that he did not find it meaningful to take notes as he feels the same way every morning. The therapist notes that he does not seem to be embarrassed about breaking their agreement. She asks him if he has any feelings about not having done what they had decided on. Arthur again seems irritated.

- I get the feeling that you're irritated. Is that so?
- Perhaps frustrated. I don't see the meaning of noting what I feel every day.
- So, you're somewhat annoyed of me asking you?
- I guess you suggest what you've been taught. Perhaps it doesn't fit me.
- Ok. – I feel a little bit confused. You accepted to do it although you probably knew that you wouldn't. Perhaps I should call it duped.
- People all the time get disappointed of me. Now that I have a depression, I think people might be a little more understanding.

Pause

- In a way I seem to blame you and you seem to do the same with me. Perhaps we should try to find out what's going on between us.
- My feeling is that you press me, that you become kind of intrusive with your attempts.-

The therapist ponders for a while. First, she tried to get Arthur to do some homework and now she wants him to comment on their relationship. She realizes that she may be seen as pushy.

- I guess you're right. It happens that I get eager to help.
- People tend to. I realize it's for my best, but I get pretty tired of it. My wife wants me to get over the fears I had about our son. But I don't know if that's the reason. I hate to have others tell me what's wrong with me. I need some space.
- So, your wife pushes you to get over the fears about your son. And I get kind of pushy. What do you feel about it?
- I don't know. I think I stop listening.

Arthur seems to go into a kind of private mental asylum. The next sessions were spent on exploring what this means to him and to what extent he is ready to invite others to his private space. The therapist tries again to talk about Arthur's worries about the child, but she gets the feeling that she ought to be careful about that. She comments several times on her cautiousness. Step by step, Arthur finds words to express that people try press feelings out of him that he has not formulated for himself yet.

The process shows how attempts to work with symptoms turned to an exploration of the patient's need protect a private part that he felt was intruded upon (Ogden, 2018; Winnicott, 1963). Important aspects of what it means to be human for Arthur were discovered in a short time: "healthy persons communicate and enjoy communicating, [but] the other fact is equally true, that each individual is an isolate, permanently non-communicating, permanently unknown, in fact unfound" (Winnicott, 1963, p. 187). A circumscribed but problematic aspect in Arthur was identified. His symptoms did not disappear, but his perspective on them changed. He left therapy with a more accepting approach to himself and possibly a new perspective of how to communicate with others.

As a metaphor, a contrast between horizontal and vertical change can be attempted. Both patients and therapists often want to reduce the extent of symptoms. This can be seen as a horizontal endeavor, a way to limit the area of symptoms. Relational therapy focuses on the vertical perspective, on the meaning of the patient's suffering. In some theories, it could be called acceptance (Hayes, Strosahl, & Wilson, 2012). A better word would be that Arthur has found and formulated new aspects of his way of being with others, and an ounce of a more meaningful relation to himself.

2 Empirical studies

There have often been tensions between practicing psychodynamic psychotherapists and psychotherapy research. Many clinicians have found research findings to be of peripheral interest for the complexity of their daily work; researchers on the other hand may consider clinicians ignorant about systematic knowledge that could make treatments more effective (Safran, Abreu, Ogilvie, & DeMaria, 2011).

The American Psychological Association's initiative for developing criteria for assessment of the scientific evidence of psychological treatments, the "evidence movement" (Chambless et al., 1996; Task Force, 1995), was met with critic and calls to honour the experience of practicing psychotherapists (APA, 2006). Nowhere in psychotherapy has the ideological distance between practice and science been more visible than between relational psychoanalysts and empirical research (Hoffman, 2009a; Lingiardi, Holmqvist, & Safran, 2016).

Despite disdain from relational psychoanalysts, empirical researchers often refer to relational theory as a theoretical base (Atzil-Slonim & Tschacher, 2020; Bernhardt, Nissen-Lie, & Råbu, 2020). New scientific analysis methods have opened for studies of processes in individual therapies and made it possible to systematically study phenomena like the alliance and corrective emotional experience minutely (Muntigl & Horvath, 2014b; Zilcha-Mano, 2019).

The basic stance in relational treatment is to understand the uniqueness of the patient and his or her suffering, to explore how the patient's psychological problems infuse the therapeutic relationship and to allow the therapeutic relationship to evolve on its own premises. In this perspective, strivings to categorize and quantify human experience seem farfetched and unreasonable.

From the opposite perspective, systematic knowledge grows from systematization of phenomena. The scientific revolution beginning in the 17th century was largely focused on categorization and quantification. Even the most unique and personal forms of human interaction can be studied as examples of general categories and processes. And they have. Psychotherapy research has shown that by using a variety of methods, intriguing and

DOI: 10.4324/9781003026914-2

clinically valuable findings can be made. The fact that the individual therapy moves in its unique way is undisputable but does not prevent the building of general knowledge, be it from case descriptions, detailed analyses of therapy dialogues or ratings of process aspects.

Some researchers assert that knowledge about psychotherapy has moved from being eminence-based to being evidence-based. The move from "As Freud wrote …" or "Winnicott found …" to replicated findings of significant phenomena is a methodological step forward. Astute clinical observation and reflective theory-building by far-sighted theorists have contributed to knowledge about psychotherapeutic processes, and not least to concepts and theoretical models. Studies of alliance ruptures and their resolutions are telling examples. In the language of science, psychoanalytic observations have had a great hypothesis-generating potential. But hypotheses must be exposed to scrutiny and to at least some form of replication.

Can the opposites of clinical observations and reflections on one hand and systematic studies on the other make a fruitful combination? It may be helpful to understand the differences between the language of science and the language of the clinician. Shahar (2010) distinguished between three forms of speaking: the pragmatic, the poetic, and the schematic. Pragmatics is everyday speech: "my car broke yesterday". Poetics are metaphors, for instance, in the psychotherapeutic dialogue, and schematics is the language of science. The crucial point here is that the poetic language of psycho-analysis, some of which was once considered scientific, should be returned to poetics (Ogden, 2018). The oedipal situation is not an issue for researchers on development, it is a useful metaphor among psychodynamic therapists to describe a human situation. No one has tried to measure the potential space, but it is an excellent way of depicturing a specific form of relational ex-perience. These psychoanalytic concepts are not explanatory, they describe feeling states, relational experiences, fantasies, and fears like poems do. Poems, like novels and visual art, often tell us more about our contemporary challenges than a row of scientific reports. But no one would think they are on the same stage as science. It would be stupid to call for replicability.

Science, however, requires knowledge that is reliable and valid in a sys-tematic sense. It may be tempting to argue "If you can count it, that ain't it" (Holsti, 1969, p. 11). Quantitative analyses based on ratings and scorings are often denigrated in contrast to qualitative, nuanced analyses of the ther-apeutic exchange. In love and friendship, experiences cannot be generalized. In science, however, they are empirical issues (Piccirillo & Rodebaugh, 2019).

The quest for effects

Although many studies indicate that patients in psychotherapy on average get better, quite a number do not (Lambert, 2013). Not more than half the patients in controlled and naturalistic studies are improved or remitted. Recent reviews suggest that treatment results may be less favourable than previous research has indicated (Cuijpers, Karyotaki, Reijnders, & Ebert, 2018).

One explanation for these meagre results could be that authorities and insurance companies prioritize a medical model with treatment packages for diagnoses ("protocol-per-syndrome"; Hofmann & Hayes, 2019) rather than personalized therapies. Mitchell (1997) argued that change comes when the therapist stops trying to find a generic method and instead fits the treatment to the unique patient. Unfortunately, psychoanalytic therapies no less than others have a tradition of trying to fit the patient to the method rather than the other way. Recent advances in psychotherapy research strongly advocate the need to understand change in a personalized way (Zilcha-Mano, 2020).

Randomized studies of psychotherapy

Understandably, psychological treatments are often studied in the same way as medical treatments. After all, most psychological treatments are delivered in publicly financed health services or with reimbursement from insurance companies or non-governmental organizations (NGOs). The issue of accountability cannot be bypassed. It is rather a question of what and how to measure (Sandell & Wilczek, 2016).

Systematic studies of psychotherapy often follow the logic of randomization and comparisons with controls. Golden standard studies are randomized; the etiquette "evidence-based" presupposes such designs. The procedure in randomized trials is to select patients randomly for different treatments, in such numbers that all significant characteristics of the participants in the two groups will be even, on average. The only feature that differs between the groups is the treatment given. This design model presumes a syndrome being treated and not a person, similarly to an antibiotic against tonsillitis. Randomizing can produce groups of persons that have the same averages on significant variables. Unique persons cannot be randomized in order to become on average equal.

The randomized trial also presumes that the treatment is the same for all patients. No one would want different ingredients in the antibiotics pill. In randomized treatments, researchers strive to make the treatment, usually delivered by different therapists, as uniform as possible. Treatment manuals are followed, adherence to them is checked.

Method comparisons

Tremendous effort has been put into clinical trials of psychotherapy. To many researchers' dismay, differences in treatment results are small when fair comparisons are made (Barber, Muran, McCarthy, & Keefe, 2013; Cuijpers, 2016; Leichsenring, Kruse, & Rabung, 2015; Leichsenring, Luyten et al., 2015; Lilliengren, Johansson, Lindqvist, Mechler, & Andersson, 2016; Lorenzo-Luaces & DeRubeis, 2018; Svensson et al., 2021). The main findings are usually that the variation between individual therapies is more impressive than differences between methods. Some treatments are successful, other produce moderate change, and some are failures. With all methods.

For some types of problems and some outcome ratings, psychodynamic therapies seem to be as favourable as other treatments, e.g. for patients with depression, with personality problems and other severe states (Driessen et al., 2015; Hofmann, Asnaani, Vonk, Sawyer, & Fang, 2012; Luyten & Blatt, 2012; Town, Abbass, & Hardy, 2011). Psychodynamic patients often improve at follow-up more than other patients (Svensson et al., 2021).

Such findings should not, however, obscure that a majority of studies show better effects for CBT therapies in routine care and in randomized trials, both with regard to symptom change and life quality (Watzke et al., 2012). There is, unfortunately, a tendency among researchers with a penchant for psychodynamic therapy to become querulous about this picture (Cornelius, 2018), sometimes by "making palliative suggestions" (Fonagy, 2010, p. 84). Arguments may be that dynamic therapy does not lend itself to the design of randomized studies, the use of treatment manuals may be inappropriate, therapists follow the process in other ways than by manuals, standard outcome measures are unfit, dynamic therapies need more experienced therapists than usually available, the therapies in trials are too short to make justice to psychoanalytic principles. These arguments are dubious (Fonagy, 2010). If researchers do attempt to make randomized trials, they should accept the rules.

Treatment integrity

A key aspect of randomized trials is reliable diagnoses and treatment manuals to check assessment and treatment integrity, that is, adherence to techniques and competence to administer them. There is a psychodynamic literature on assessment and treatment in relation to diagnoses (e.g. McWilliams, 1999, 2004; Operationalized Psychodynamic Diagnosis, 2008), and some researchers argue for more structured dynamic therapies that can be studied rigorously. Fonagy (2010) suggested that therapists should practice a "loose manualisation of routine psychodynamic treatment" (p. 84).

The idea that treatments should be constructed for syndromes, with identical patients and identical treatments (the uniformity myths), similarly to medical therapies, has been criticized for many years (Kiesler, 1966). Although cherished by authorities, this design model has been questioned by researchers with different perspectives (Hofmann & Hayes, 2019; Insel et al., 2010; Johnstone & Boyle, 2018).

Research overviews generally fail to find support for the value of treatment adherence for outcome (Truijens et al., 2019; Webb, DeRubeis, & Barber, 2010). The idea of guidelines is foreign to relational theories. Therapeutic stances are based on theoretical understanding rather than specific techniques. The emphasis not only on the unique patient but also on the unique patient-therapist dyad makes relational therapy particularly unsuited for standardization.

But although this perspective is commendable, it should not be denied that it is also a problem in times of demands of public accountability. It may be true that "exclusive reliance on one technique appears to be a correlate of inexperience" (Strupp, 1955, p. 7). But not all therapists are experienced, not all are even good enough. The task of delivering person-centred treatment in a public climate of justified claims for accountability is a challenge.

The common relational factors

In psychotherapy research, there has for a long time been a debate between proponents of the idea that specific techniques are the main change factors, and the notion that factors common to most methods, mostly relational, have a stronger importance for outcome. This discussion started in 1936 when Saul Rosenzweig suggested that most therapies give equal results, and that the reason may be that there are common factors in therapies that account for most of the effect, rather than their specific techniques. His paper was the start of two major strands of thought that have been extremely important and much debated in psychotherapy research. The "dodo bird verdict" states that average differences in outcome between therapies are small for most conditions and treatments. This view has on the whole been corroborated by current research (Lambert, 2013; Lorenzo-Luaces & DeRubeis, 2018; Wampold & Imel, 2015). The other assertion, that treatment outcome is due to factors common to most methods more than to techniques specific to methods, is still strongly debated (Baker & McFall, 2014; Frank & Frank, 1993; Rogers, 1957; Wampold & Imel, 2015).

The common factors perspective says that relational factors and characteristics, either in the therapist (Rogers, 1957), in the patient (Beutler et al., 2018), or in the emergent interplay between patient and therapist (Horvath, 2018; Safran & Muran, 2000), are the decisive factors for therapeutic success. An apparent problem in this discussion is the difficulty to make distinctions between techniques and relational interventions. Where is the border between active work with alliance ruptures as a technique and the general focus on collaboration and alliance reparation in all therapies? Which therapist would not, more or less explicitly, challenge the patient to meet anxiety-provoking situations? In which treatment is not mirroring, sometimes called validation, used? In a fruitful therapy, the therapist may decide to use a common factor, like empathy, in a focused and systematic way. Is it still a common factor?

Another problem in making studies of causal relations between common factors and outcome is that the common factors often are aspects of the therapist's or the patient's personality, or of the emergent interaction. It is impossible to randomly assign factors like therapist empathy and warmth, patient motivation and expectations, or a collaborative atmosphere to different groups of therapies. We know that there is a statistical correlation between patients' alliance ratings and symptom change from session to session (Zilcha-Mano, 2019)? But how do we know that factors that co-vary with alliance do not cause the potential change?

Although still vital among therapists and the general public, the common factors dispute has largely been superseded among researchers by more intricate and complex models of therapeutic change focusing on the interdependence of common and specific factors (Cuijpers, Reijnders, & Huibers, 2019; de Felice et al., 2019). A viable alliance does not arise in the same way in a relation-focused therapy as in a solution-focused treatment (Tschacher, Junghan, & Pfammatter, 2012). Relational therapy is an obvious example of how so-called common factors are used as technique, tailor-made for each patient.

The therapeutic relationship

The therapeutic relationship is the focus of relational therapy. It is also to a large extent the focus of psychotherapy research. Interactional studies can be made with different degrees of granularity. On the most finely calibrated level, line by line studies use *conversation analysis* (Keselman, Osvaldsson Cromdal, Kullgard, & Holmqvist, 2018; Peräkylä, 2019; Viklund, Holmqvist, & Zetterqvist Nelson, 2010; Voutilainen & Peräkylä, 2016). Vehviläinen (2003), for instance, studied how therapists turn the patient's narrative into useful therapeutic stories (see also Antaki, 2008; Antaki, Barnes, & Leudar, 2005). Other lines of research have analysed how patients handle situations to avoid open conflict with medical doctors (Heath, 1992; Heritage & Clayman, 2010) as well as with their psychotherapists (Muntigl & Horvath, 2014a; Viklund et al., 2010).

Empirical research has shown the fruitfulness of exploring maladaptive interactional patterns in the relationship with the therapist (Dinger, Zilcha-Mano, McCarthy, Barrett, & Barber, 2013; Mikulincer, Shaver, & Berant, 2013). Many methods also study interactional recurrent patterns outside the therapy relationship (Benjamin, 1996; Kiesler, 1986; Young et al., 2003). From a psychoanalytic perspective, it is sometimes argued that these methods provoke intellectualized rather than genuine emotional work (Gabbard & Westen, 2003).

In psychoanalysis, the therapy relationship is usually described as aspects of transference and countertransference. The empirical research on transference is limited (Crits-Christoph & Gibbons, 2002; Høglend & Gabbard, 2012). Studies show various results; several of them suggest that transference interpretations may be negative for process and outcome (McCullough et al., 1991). Høglend et al. (2006), 2008 found that therapies using transference interpretations and therapies without such interpretations had similar results; however, patients with poor real-life relationships fared better in therapies using transference interpretations, suggesting that transference work may have more of a skills training value than usually thought. Based on the mixed findings, Luyten (2015) argues that therapists should be cautious about the risks of negative effects of transference interpretations.

The alliance

The alliance is one aspect of the therapeutic relationship; it is the collaborative side of it (Hatcher & Barends, 2006). Rooted in Freud's idea of the "friendly and affectionate aspects of the transference which are admissible to consciousness, and which are the vehicle of success" (Freud, 1912b, p. 105), Sterba (1934) was the first to use the concept alliance for cooperation in therapy. Later, Zetzel (1956) used "therapeutic alliance" for the emotional aspect of the cooperation and Greenson (1965) "working alliance" for cooperation on the therapeutic tasks. Luborsky (1976) described the "helping alliance" as a combination of the patient's idea of the therapist as a helpful and competent person and the patient's commitment to the common work.

Alliance is cooperation. It is not a method; it is an aspect of how the method is used (Hatcher & Barends, 2006). When cooking together, it is nice to cooperate. But no one would think that cooperation by itself gives any meals. Cooperation around the cooking may make the meal better. A symphony concert needs musicians who cooperate while they play. Better cooperation makes better music.

Current research underlines two aspects of the alliance as important for outcome. One is its strength; better alliance, as reported by both patient and therapist, leads to better outcome (Flückiger, Del Re, Wampold, & Horvath, 2018). This is valid also for session-to-session associations; stronger alliance in one session is associated with symptom reduction in the next (Flückiger et al., 2020).

The other aspect is fluctuations, impasses, ruptures, and the therapeutic work to repair them. Bordin (1994) argued that alliance is a process, attempts to restore the alliance is natural and an aspect of its usefulness in therapy. Safran and Muran (2000) describe therapeutic work on alliance problems as a way to explore and modify patients' dysfunctional interpersonal schemas. In this view, work on the alliance is part of the therapeutic method.

These two perspectives on the therapeutic utility of the alliance are obviously similar to the psychoanalytic idea of the relationship as containing both uncontroversial positive aspects and transferential elements reflecting the patient's troubled relational expectations.

Ruptures and resolution processes

Relational theory as well as empirical research have taken a large interest in alliance ruptures and how to repair them (Muran, 2019). Studies show that therapies where the therapist detects alliance problems and address them have better outcome (Chen et al., 2018). Therapists often do not detect discontent among their patients (Eubanks, Muran & Safran, 2019; Rhodes, Hill, Thompson, & Elliot, 1994) although observers may find ruptures in almost all sessions (Eubanks et al., 2019). Even experienced therapists to a large extent miss their patients' negative feelings (Hill, Thompson, Cogar, & Denman, 1993), often because patients are not able or ready to disclose when they feel uncomfortable or disagree with their therapist (Hill, 2010).

In all therapy models, therapists are taught to detect alliance problems, and to resolve them in order to avoid poor treatment adherence and premature termination. The specific point in relational therapy is that resolutions of ruptures are seen as curative interventions (Muntigl & Horvath, 2014b). Rupture is a strong word. Sometimes, confrontative ruptures shake the therapist, put the therapy in danger. The patient may show discontent with the treatment, the mutual work, the therapist, the results. But more often, rupture denotes embroilments, troubles, tangles, hassles, and pettifogging. Or withdrawal, lack of interest, disengagement. Subtle hardly noticeable problems (Safran, Muran, & Eubanks-Carter, 2011). "Because the process of chaining relational moves together (sometimes very loosely) is largely spontaneous and unpredictable from one move to the next, there are many mismatches, derailments, misunderstandings, and indeterminacies. These 'mistakes' require a process of repair" (Stern, 2004b, p. 368). The focus on the relationship process, comprising fluctuations due to contributions from both therapist and patient, may be the point where psychoanalytic theories and empirical research can find common ground. Process, rather than states and traits, may be a common denominator.

3 The road to the relational perspective

Relational psychoanalytic therapy is an amalgam of different theories and influences. The publication of Greenberg's and Mitchell's "Object relations in psychoanalytic theory" (1983) was the starting point for a movement that had germinated for some time among primarily interpersonal psychoanalysts in the United States. Time was ripe for a combination of the interpersonal psychoanalytic tradition with influences from the British object-relations tradition, the self-psychological perspective, and a general movement towards more open and creative ways to use the therapeutic relationship.

Many among the relational originators came from the interpersonal tradition, inspired by Sullivan and by European psychoanalysts like Erich Fromm, Clara Thompson, Karen Horney, and Frieda Fromm-Reichmann. These arrived in the United States during the 1930s and developed their unique versions of culture-sensitive psychoanalytic ideas. After harsh disputes between interpersonalists, often trained at the William Alanson White Institute in New York, and orthodox analysts during several decades, the relational turn came as a liberating force, with great enthusiasm and a strong impact on psychoanalytic theory development (Stern, 2015).

Relational therapy as an identified movement was born in a specific time period, the 1980s, among culturally liberal psychoanalysts in New York and other American cities. The intellectual climate was coloured by the radical cultural and political movements in the Western world in the 1960s and 1970s (Seligman, 2019). Protests against the Vietnam war and the Civil Rights movement were a fertile ground for upheaval of traditional values and structures. From these general cultural roots, the relational movement brought an anti-authoritarian attitude, a critical perspective on traditional gender and sexual roles, a quest for authenticity, and an eagerness for improvisation and spontaneity (Safran, 2017).

Looking back 50 plus years, there has been a radical change in psychoanalytic theory from ideas of innate drives and fantasies to an emphasis on the relational underpinnings of human life (Aron & Leichich, 2012; Fonagy & Campbell, 2015). This road has passed through Fairbairn's idea of a primary drive towards relationships, object relations theories, attachment theory, and mentalization theory. New concepts such as mirroring (Kohut,

DOI: 10.4324/9781003026914-3

1971), holding (Winnicott, 1971b), containment (Bion, 1962), and sensitive responding (Ainsworth, Blehar, Waters, & Wall, 1978) have altered the view not only of the background of patients' problems but also about how to help them. Meta-psychological theories are on decline. Instead of creating models of the structure of the mind, psychodynamic psychotherapists have moved to a greater interest in therapeutic processes, seeing them as a narrative project, a rebuilding of attachment trust, or as a way to explore new relational possibilities (Mitchell, 1988; Schafer, 1983).

In all revolutions, there is a risk that new ideas get stuck in their own wheel tracks, that they become institutionalized (Wachtel, 2018). Relational is a prestige word in contemporary psychotherapy, but the specific ideas of the relational psychoanalytic movement and their therapeutic implications are not well known in wider psychotherapeutic circles. One reason could be that relational theorists, although generally open to different influences, are wary of combining their ideas with other psychotherapeutic orientations. Wachtel (2018) observed that although relational theory has been considered to be both integrative (Aron, 1996) and rebellious, its proponents have stopped short of integrating their ideas with other therapy orientations.

The conceptual underpinnings

Relational theory can easily be perceived as a labyrinth of ideas and models. In an attempt to create a comprehensive model, and to connect relational thoughts with older relational theories, Mitchell (1988, 2000) suggested a relational matrix with three dimensions; the self, the other, and the interaction between them. According to him, earlier theorists with relational perspectives have emphasized one of these dimensions. Theories where the coherence of the self has a primary place, like Kohut's and Winnicott's, are *relational by implication*. These models presuppose a cohesive self. The self is born from the holding or mirroring safety offered by the caregiver. The models are relational in the sense that they suggest that the individual's self grows in interaction with a caregiver or therapist. Development of the "authentic", "true" self (Winnicott, 1965) comes through the therapist's reparative activities.

Theories that emphasize the individual's striving for contact, the need of an object, are *relational by intent*. Fairbairn (1952) and Fromm are examples. In their theories, the individual longs for the other, and has a drive for relationship, also when the relationship is destructive. These theories put emphasis on how relationships create the inner world of the patient, on the formation of residues of object relations in the individual. Fairbairn's selfobject units are examples, replacing the "seething cauldron" in the id with different variants of self-object constellations.

Bowlby (1969) and Sullivan (1953) represent the *relational by design* dimension, meaning that humans are constructed to live in relationships, that the relationship is the basis for understanding a person. Sullivan's statement that "personality can never be isolated from the complex of interpersonal relations" (Sullivan, 1953, p. 10) is an expression of this standpoint. These theories focus on the actual, here-and-now interaction in the therapeutic interaction. "What's going on around here" is a classical description of this therapeutic stance (Levenson & Feiner, 1991). The research made by the Boston CPSG (2010) is typical of this view, underlining the implicit, ongoing relating in the therapeutic relationship as curative.

The conflict perspective

In its Freudian guise, psychoanalytic thinking has focused on conflicts between conscious and preconscious experiences on one hand, and repressed, unconscious mental content on the other. Psychological problems and, indeed, our whole life are made up of conflicting conceptions, emotions, thoughts, and ideas, largely unconscious to us (Brenner, 1982). The focus of interpretative therapy is to make the patient aware of how problematic behaviours, symptoms, and beliefs are expressions of repressed desires and feelings. Modern affect-focused dynamic therapies often rely on this drive (emotion) conflict model.

Relational conflict

An important expression of unconscious, repressed memories is the patient's distorted notions of the therapist, that is, the transference. In the transference, the intrapsychic becomes interpersonal; the mental world is projected on the therapeutic situation. By taking a neutral stance, the therapist can help the patient reflect on distinctions between distortions and veridical views of the relationship.

With a constructivist perspective on therapy, the understanding of the relational interplay entails that both participants contribute to the interaction. Transference is always coloured by countertransference. The therapist's unavoidable and unwitting participation in dyadic enactments makes shared curiosity the reasonable stance. The focus is on exploring co-created, new possibilities in the interpersonal field (Stern, 2015). The everyday illustration of this model is two partners getting into conflict. If one of them purports to discover repressed intentions in the other's mind, the discussion will probably not end well. But if both are open to exploring their own contributions to the conflict, they may find new ways of being together.

Models of the mind

Psychoanalytic theories present a conflicted mind. Memories, intentions, painful experiences, and forbidden fantasies are kept in the dark, out of awareness. Even the capacity to create knowledge may be destroyed (Bion, 1962). In these models, the subjective core self is unitary.

The relational model of the mind opens for multiples selves. The self is a combination of more or less dissociated self-states. The subject changes over time and situations, using and creating self-states for contextual reasons. In theory, there may be as many personalities as there are interpersonal contexts (Sullivan, 1940). Mental spaces that are inaccessible, unavailable, without meaning or affective intensity limit personal development.

The idea that the individual is organized as configurations of multiple self-states (Bromberg, 1998; Slavin, 1996) implies that the idea of a core or true self is inadequate. Varying self-other configurations, tied together with affects, in patient and therapist, meet each other. Bromberg used the felicitous expression *standing in the spaces* to describe the ability to be aware of different aspects of oneself, to tolerate ambiguity and uncertainty with regard to who I "really" am.

Transference and countertransference

Transference interpretation is the cornerstone of psychoanalytic technique. The idea of the neutral, anonymous, and abstinent therapist who stimulates transference manifestations has had a long life in the psychoanalytic tradition, often exaggerated, considering that Freud's contacts with his patients were neither neutral nor abstinent (Roazen, 1995).

Even if transference interpretations are made tentatively, the one-person perspective by principle means that the therapist has the privilege and the responsibility to suggest interpretations about the patient's mental world, particularly aspects that are not conscious to the patient. During the past decades, psychodynamic therapists have largely rejected the model of the therapist as a blank screen. In reality, transference work has probably for a long time been considered as a mutual enterprise. "Every psychoanalyst unavoidably works upon his own fantasies on the basis of those he hears from his patients and works upon their fantasies on the basis of his own" wrote Roustang in 1976. Baranger, Baranger, and Mom (1983) called it a "shared fantasy". Still most traditional dynamic therapists probably try to follow a pragmatic line and work as if the patient's reactions on the whole can be seen as reflecting recurrent patterns.

Countertransference

Since the first days of psychoanalysis the question of how the counter-transference, that is, the therapist's reactions to the patient, should be handled has been in focus. When Freud's first co-worker Joseph Breuer – we are in the 1880s – realized that his patient Anna O thought she was pregnant with him, he went on vacation with his wife on a second honeymoon. During this holiday Breuer's third child was conceived. Was that a way for Breuer to keep away unwanted wishes and fears? It seems like a riddle as Anna O was not pregnant and Breuer knew that. They had (most likely) not been intimate with each other. Did he nonetheless have a need to keep undesired fantasies at a distance?

The description is given by Freud in a letter to Stefan Zweig many years after the incident. The fascinating thing in the story is that Freud's description is not true. Breuer went on a planned vacation with his family, wife, and children. Their last child was born several months earlier. Freud created the story from his memory and fantasies. In this construction of a story about the therapist's troubled reactions, Freud shows the strong emotional loading in the therapist's and even the therapist's colleague's feelings and fantasies evoked by intensive therapeutic work.

All therapists react to their patients. The question is what place these reactions should take in the understanding of the therapeutic interplay. During the first decades of psychoanalysis, countertransference was perceived as a problem for the therapist (Freud, 1910). Countertransference was considered to be the therapist's transference, to be remedied by personal analysis and supervision, but with no relevance for the understanding of the patient.

Interest in the therapeutic value of the countertransference started to grow around 1950 among psychoanalysts of different schools. Winnicott (1949) wrote about the "objective countertransference", meaning specific emotional reactions that all therapists would have towards a certain patient. Heimann (1950) suggested that the countertransference may be the patient's creation, meaning the patient's way of engendering distinct reactions in the therapist. Bion (1962) used the Kleinian concept "projective identification" to describe how the patient deposits unconscious and disavowed material in the therapist, evoking feelings that are felt as unfamiliar to her. The question "does the anger come from you or from your patient" was considered meaningful.

Another influence on the understanding of countertransference came from the American interpersonal tradition. Searles, for instance, argued that one cause for a patient's psychotic defense is that he has sensed his parent's serious mental troubles but been forbidden to comment on them (Searles, 1975). When the same thing happens in therapy, it is the therapist's responsibility to disclose that the patient's perception has some truth in it. It is an extreme form of self-disclosure, in a way parallel to what Ferenczi tried in the early 1930s. The countertransference is in this view not a reaction to the patient, it is a discovery by the patient.

Some empirical studies have been made of therapists' reported feelings towards patients. Tanzilli, Muzi, Rønningstam, and Lingiardi (2017) found that narcissistic patients evoked hostile, devalued, inadequate, and disengaged feelings; Colli, Tanzilli, Dimaggio, and Lingiardi (2014) found that borderline patients evoked helpless, overwhelmed, and overinvolved feelings in therapists; and Holmqvist and Armelius (2004) found that borderline patients who evoked negative, angry, and rejected feelings had better outcome at follow-up.

However, these studies of "objective countertransference" do not answer the relational question of the usefulness of countertransference feelings in individual therapies. Using the two-person perspective, the question is not if the countertransference gives information about the patient but if it is useful for mutual exploration of the interplay. The challenge is: "how do we offer patients our own understandings of what might be happening between us as a collaborative endeavor that enhances rather than undermines mutual recognition and self-growth?" (Davies, 2018, p. 660).

Immediacy

The relational conception of work in the therapeutic relationship focuses on experiences rather than representations. Representational work implies an interest in how the patient's image of the therapist and the therapeutic relationship successively is colored by the patient's internalized relational patterns. As these representations become conscious and possible to verbalize, they can be used for interpretations about the patient's life. With this approach, the *content* of the transference-countertransference relationship is in focus.

Work on experiences, on the *process*, in the relationship focuses on the ongoing affective interaction, on immediate feelings and moods. Described from the therapist's perspective, it may sound like this:

– Suddenly I had the impression that we are talking about something more solemn than I first thought. I guess I would call my feeling awe. Do you feel anything like that?

This is an observation about a change in the interactional atmosphere. The therapist does not try mind reading; she starts in her own mind. The focus is on the feeling, not on the representational aspect of the dialog. The dialog might continue like this:

– I have heard that before. People seem to become awed about what I made in the refugee camp. But there wasn't anything else for me to do. I couldn't just leave the others. It wouldn't have been possible to continue living with the thought that I had abandoned them.
– I felt impressed by your courage. But you seem more occupied by the responsibility aspect.
– People exaggerate what I did. Most people would have done the same.
– I am thinking I get the feeling that what I felt as impressive was in some way trivial for you.
– Well, perhaps not trivial but it's hard to understand, perhaps it's hard for me to take.
– You mean the praise? I just thought about it. Like I lifted you up in a way that didn't feel comfortable to you.

The therapist tries to capture the ongoing emotional process. There are sources in the patient's (and in the therapist's) life for the reactions. But the gauge is the emotional loading. It should also be noticed that the therapist's comment does not target a conflict. The "conflict" ensues after the comment, in this instance rather as an incongruence.

The focus on immediate emotional experiences in the therapeutic relationship means that interest in associations with repressed memories from previous relationships ("genetic transference interpretations") has decreased. Although it may be natural for both patient and therapist to make such reflections, they do not always contribute to therapeutic change. They may even be considered as mutual resistance, when they imply a "return to the past, to the quieter historical and narrative aspects of the psychodynamics. The relationship as it exists in the here and now is abandoned and the treatment continues on another plane" (Stern, 2004a, s. 140).

Focus on the immediate interaction has various purposes. Basically, it opens up for reflections on the ongoing interaction, offering an observational perspective. Often, it heightens the affective temperature by focusing on the interaction. Sometimes, it contributes to new, reconstructive experiences. Seen in this way, the relationship has a relationally reparative function rather than being targeted on insight. "the therapeutic encounter provides a protected testing ground for experimenting with new ways of thinking, feeling, and relating. Focusing on the in-session affective and relational experiences ... might serve as a template for new adaptive relational experiences in the patient's life" (DeFife, Hilsenroth, & Kuutmann, 2015, p. 523).

4 Problems in relating

The intertwining between psychoanalytic theory, clinical experience, and research on infants' development has a century-long tradition. Freud's early ideas were speculative and based on theoretical assumptions and clinical hunches from the treatment of adult patients. Concepts like "the anal phase" or "the oedipal situation" were once considered as empirical descriptions but have retreated to theoretical conceptualization and clinical parlance (Fonagy, Target, & Gergely, 2006; Govrin, 2016). Since the ground-breaking observational studies of Mahler, Pine, and Bergman (1973) and Ainsworth, Blehar, Waters, and Wall (1978), systematic empirical research on early development has enriched the understanding of the interplay in the therapeutic interaction.

Developmental studies have significance in two ways in relational therapy. One is to trace origins of adult problems to childhood experiences. The other is to understand how the principles governing interplay between caregivers and children can shed light on the therapeutic interplay.

Attachment

Attachment theory has a significant place in current psychoanalytic thinking as a way of understanding aspects of the therapy and as a potential goal for treatment.

The attachment model implies that recurrent experiences in childhood become engraved as internal working models, influencing current ways of relating. Studies have confirmed the association between early attachment patterns and later interpersonal behaviour, but also brought nuances to the model (Groh et al., 2017; van Ijzendoorn & Bakermans-Kranenburg, 2008; Verhage et al., 2016). The idea of consistent attachment patterns ("internal working models") has been questioned conceptually and empirically in recent years (Luyten, 2015).

Several studies have, for instance, suggested that the genetic influence on attachment patterns may be larger than previously thought (Fearon, Shmueli-Goetz, Viding, Fonagy, & Plomin, 2014; Fraley & Roberts, 2005; Tucker-Drob & Briley, 2019).

DOI: 10.4324/9781003026914-4

When researchers started observing infant-child interactions, they soon found that attachment development is a mutual process. Infants are active very early in relating to their caregivers. "We begin life 'connected,' as part of each other ... We begin in relationship" (Sander, 2008, p. 170). The child's reality is a shared: "Infant research teaches us that human external reality is inherently shared because it is constructed out of shared feeling, shared intentions, and shared plans" (Fonagy & Target, 2007, p. 921; see also Beebe, Knoblauch, Rustin, & Sorter, 2005; Fonagy, Gergely, Jurist, & Target, 2002).

The parent's affective attunement to the child's mental state, and the child's reciprocal ability to evoke attunement in the parent, are central to the child's development. Subtle changes in muscle tone, shifts in vocalization, changes in body posture, contours of movements influence the other (Beebe et al., 2005; Downing, 2006; Stern, 2004). Attunement is cross-modal; perception of the child's rhythmical speech can make the caregiver respond with rhythmically touching the child (Beebe et al., 2005; Stern, 1984, 1985). The emotional atmosphere, encompassing vitality affects as well as categorical affects, is central for the development of secure attachment (Beebe et al., 2010, 2012).

Relationship breaches

Detailed relational exploration of subtle or not so subtle ruptures and ways to resolve them lie at the heart of relational therapy. The "Still face" situation (Tronick, 1989) shows how the child's desperate need to remain in contact with his caregiver evokes the caregiver's wish to repair the contact rupture. The ways of resolving contact breaches are unique for each parent–child dyad. Some children have to find ways to engage parents who disappear in smartphones or look downhearted on the wall; every child finds ways to catch the parent's attention, or to find ways to tolerate the lack of it.

Tronick and Cohn (1989) found in studies of face-to-face interaction that states of incongruence happen in two thirds of the time. The mother may, for instance, be eager to play while the child just attends to what is going on. Most ruptures and the repairs of them are quite subtle and fast; in 70% of the unmatched states, repair occurred within two seconds. These recurring experiences of repair of ruptures are fundamental to the child's experience of the interaction.

The child's trust in his ability to repair mismatches enhances his feelings of relational competence (Beebe & Lachmann, 2013; Tronick & Cohn, 1989). In attachment building dialogues, the expectation develops that it is possible to maintain engagement with the partner despite strains and mismatches (Beebe & Lachmann, 1994). Studies of intersubjective systems underline the importance of the child's learning how to handle "messy" interactions (Sander, 2008; Trevarthen, 1979). "mismatches of affective states, miscoordination of responses, and misapprehensions of relational intentions" is the normal way of relating (Ham & Tronick, 2009, p. 620).

Relational competence

Mental health problems are associated with relational deadlocks and dysfunctions. Problems evolving from constitutional influences and life history become expressed and experienced in the individual's relationships. In comparison with other mammals, human beings' relational competence is less genetically determined and to a larger extent dependent on learning from caregivers (Fonagy, Luyten, & Allison, 2015).

The emphasis on constitutional and life historical factors changes over time in psychiatry. The trend over the past decades has been to focus on genetic and other biological factors (Harrington, 2019). Schizophrenia, bipolar disorder, ADHD, and autism are nowadays usually seen as mainly genetically grounded, although causal neurological and genetical indicators are hard to find.

The balance between constitutional and life historical perspectives has significance for how to work with the patient. Emphasis on brain dysfunction has often bred pessimism regarding radical cure (Kvaale, Haslam, & Gottdiener, 2013; Pescosolido et al., 2010). When neurological dysfunction is considered to be the main cause of problems, treatment efforts become focused on education and adaptation. The individual will need to understand his functional dysfunction and its consequences.

A broader interest in the neurological underpinnings of social behaviour is offered by social neuroscience, studies of neurologically imposed limitations and possibilities of social competence (Cacioppo & Berntson, 1992). "Deficits in any one of these component processes can result in personal difficulties and interpersonal problems that are prominent features in a variety of mental disorders" (Cacioppo, Cacioppo, & Dulawa, 2014, p. 131). Although usually one-directional: mapping the influence of the brain on social behaviour and experience, there has also been an interest in the structural impact of life experiences like traumas on the brain (Siegel, 2001).

From a treatment perspective, neuroscience has up till now contributed very few therapy advances for patients. Frances (2016) argued that despite the enormous progress in understanding brain function, no single patient has been helped by it to this day.

Autism

An interesting and challenging example of how to use relational therapy is the case of autism, a state with surmised neurological causes influencing behaviour and experience. A key symptom in autism is problems in social interaction, implying decreased ability to mentalize and to understand the implicit meaning in verbal communication. The general problem has been described as lack of central cognitive coherence, implying a tendency to stay in details without understanding the overarching context (Frith 2008). Although criticized, this idea gives a good idea of how to understand the functioning of autistic persons. Relationally, they usually find it easier to handle formal interactions than those that have loose structure and lack of defined goals.

A common pedagogical strategy in schools is to use pictures and cartoons, "image support", and other concrete tools. Is it meaningful and feasible to use such or similar tools in relational therapy?

Peter was successful at school. He had a degree in engineering from a prestige university. His parents were proud of him, and he was indeed clever. However, due to his start-up problems, they often helped him with his home tasks. After his studies, he had neither worked nor studied. At 28, he got the diagnosis autism. He decided to try relational therapy for his depression, inactivity, and compulsive habit of finding women for one-night stands. In therapy, he presented himself as a person interested in arts and culture. For a while, his therapist was attracted by high-brow discussions until she realized that this was no way for the patient to change his life. She tried to engage Peter in attempts to plan his days and activities. They also tried to understand the reason for Peter's compulsive need to show his sexual prowess with women. Although they understood some antecedents in previous failures with women, nothing changed, and the dialogue felt barren.

The therapist tried to talk about her feeling at her wits end in her attempts to come further. Peter felt bewildered and frustrated. He wondered whether she criticized him or if she wanted to end the therapy. She tried to explain that her intention was to invite to reflection about their interaction. Peter became angry and felt criticized for not making progress. The therapist tried to explain her reason for discussing the therapy process, but she got the feeling that Peter had stopped listening.

The therapist decided to try another way. Using her whiteboard, she concretely demonstrated with circles and arrows her view of their dialogue during the last sessions. Peter became occupied with finding faults in her drawing. She invited to him to draw himself. He agreed and made his own drawings. The comparison between the drawings proved to be a way to compare perspectives on what had taken place between them. After this, the technique could be used also to understand how Peter interacted in other relationships.

5　Theoretical principles

Two-person psychology

Relational is a buzzword in several disciplines. Philosophers Baumann (2000), Giddens (1991), and Taylor (1989) have developed theories about the relational and "situated" nature of human knowledge. Relational psychotherapy can be seen as a part of the postmodern project, where constructionism replaces positivism (Hoffman, 1998). It is, however, important not to lose the complexities in the clinical situation in attempts to use philosophical concepts for understanding the intricate interplay in the therapy relationship.

Two-person psychology or the two-person perspective is foundational for relational therapy (Aron, 1996; Ghent, 1989; Mitchell, 2000; Rickman, 1957). The concept implies not only that the interaction is mutually created; it also means that the understanding of the ongoing interaction is a mutual construction.

Many psychoanalytically based theories contend that psychological problems develop in relationships. The early trauma theory (Breuer & Freud, 1895) put a causal emphasis on troubled relational interactions with others. Likewise, Ferenczi (1933) and Balint (1968) saw problematic interactions as the roots of psychological problems. Sullivan's interpersonal psychology is an evident example of a relational perspective as is the attachment model.

However, despite their focus on the relationship, they are not two-person theories. Two-person psychology is an epistemological concept, it is about how understanding is created (Hoffman, 1983, 1998). An important step towards this position was the transition from the search for historical truth in the patient's material to the idea that the goal of therapy is to provide a more meaningful life narrative (Spence, 1982). Although the narrative model still conceives the patient as creator of his history, this perspective allows for cooperation between patient and therapist in the moulding of the patient's narrative.

The next step was when theorists realized that the mutually developed understanding is inevitably co-created, that the therapist's perspective has a

DOI: 10.4324/9781003026914-5

fundamental influence on the understanding of the patient's situation (Renik, 1993).

Let us consider this clinical situation:

The patient starts therapy because he feels depressed. Based on his history, the therapist thinks he fears intimacy with women. At one session he talks about a woman he has met. He was not romantically interested in her, but he accepted when she asked him to join her at a concert. He thought she was an expert on the kind of music that would be performed, and he wanted to hear what she thought of it. On the way to the concert hall, she proposed that they should take a drink. After the concert, they went to a café. He was keen on hearing what she thought about the performance. When they had talked for a while, he realized that she did not know very much about music. The therapist suggests that she might have been interested in his company rather than the music. He is uncertain. When asked if he was in any way flattered by her invitation, he was hesitant.

After a month, the patient invites another woman for dinner because she is a friend of his sister. They dine. Afterwards he is disappointed of her. He thinks she was pushy about becoming more friendly than he wanted. The therapist remembers the concert evening. She wonders what happened with that woman and her interest in him.

–   Was she interested in me? I thought it was the music.
–   I guess it was, but I think you said that she was keen on seeing you. She wanted to go to a bar with you.
–   Yes, perhaps she was. She sent me a card afterwards. Perhaps she wanted more contact.
–   I had the impression that you were in some way ambivalent to her, that you had some feelings but were uncertain about what you wanted.
–   I may have been.
–   As I remember it, you were somewhat curious about her, but perhaps also uncertain.
–   I wonder if you exaggerate my ambivalence about women. For the moment, I don't feel I have that kind of interest in them.

The therapist feels caught when she realizes that she may be too eager when talking about his potential interest in women. They stay for a while in the patient's reactions on women that, in his mind, are too pushy. How is the understanding of the patient's feelings for the women construed? Who turns the questions, the comments in new directions? What is a reasonable interpretation, a guess, or even a misunderstanding? The therapist thinks that the patient has a greater interest than he acknowledges and that he puts up a naïve face. It could be true. But it also makes sense that the patient's way of talking of women attracts the interest of the therapist.

There is an extensive research literature showing that therapists reformulate and reconceptualize the material that the patient brings to the session (Davis,

1986; Peräkylä, 2019). Usually unbeknownst, the therapist adjusts the direction of the conversation in alignment with her theoretical, clinical, personal, and pragmatic considerations. Relational therapy is based on the understanding that the therapist's perspective is as subjective as the patient's. The road from immediate perception to conscious reflection goes through interpretation using the conceptual and semantic tools available, the "discourses". Discourses are organized and usually unquestioned ways of using thought models and language to form and transmit knowledge and practices (Foucault, 1979, 1980). They are carriers of knowledge by providing "deeply entrenched convictions and explanatory schemas fundamental to the dominant form of making sense of the world" (Sawicki, 1991, p. 104). In the relational epistemological model, the participants bring their discursive resources to the relationship, but they also successively develop a dyadic discourse specific for them.

Two-person psychology is an epistemological discovery, but it is also a choice of perspective. Our understanding of social reality is based on gender, age, social class, and education, and also on more specific, contextually situated social and relational discourses. This is an insight that is valid for all human interaction. We can choose to ignore this knowledge. Sometimes, it is wise to keep it in the background. A physician with an emergency case may be aware of the patient's gender, age, ethnic background, and social class, and she may realize that this may have bearings on how the patient will understand a hospital treatment. But in the emergency room, she concentrates on the heart attack. A behaviour therapist treating an elevator phobia may also focus on the task at hand. But as soon as the therapeutic task targets the patient's emotional and relational problems, the question of co-creating understanding becomes relevant.

Two-person psychology and enactments

When vitality and openness in the interaction changes to a complementary doer-done-to relationship, a mutual enactment has occurred (Jacobs, 1991; Lyons-Ruth, 1999). Dyadic enactment means that patient and therapist end up in a situation where their mental mobility and creativity is limited. Understanding becomes one-dimensional instead of multifaceted and stimulating. The patient and the therapist become "hopelessly defined by the other and incapable of escaping the force of the interactive pull to act in creative and fully agentic ways" (Davies, 2003, pp. 15–16).

Enactments are defensive deletions and distortions of potential ways of understanding a relational situation. They are expressions of dyadic resistance (McLaughlin, 1991). Exploration of enactments offers a perspective on the patient–therapist dyad's difficulty and unwillingness to open for new perspectives on their relationship and on their own experience (Slochower, 2020) and is an important learning occasion.

Enactments occur in all interactions. They are not only storms or radiant sunshine but rather like clouds on ordinary days (Mitchell, 1997). Patient and therapist regularly end up in dyadic enactments that become part of their shared habitual, sometimes constrained, interaction. They express the "present unconscious" rather than "past unconscious" (Sandler & Sandler, 1994). The oscillation between different variants of dyadic modes, particularly enactments and moments experienced as potential space, is the typical process in relational therapy. Enactments are often not conscious to the participants; the feeling of deadlock or stagnation is not always perceptible (Lyons-Ruth, 1999). Consider the old couple stuck in their old ruts who is visited by their rarely seen child who says: "Why do you bicker all the time?" or "Why do you never speak seriously with each other?" They had not noticed it.

An illustration:

Peter had frequent panic attacks and feared he had some dangerous illness. He could not understand the reason for his attacks; they had started without warning and without apparent reason. He had tried medication without success and had been persuaded to try psychotherapy. He was openly sceptical but thought he might give it a try. His therapist was anxious to show that therapy might be effective, challenged by his resistance. She suggested interoceptive exposure. They tried several exercises. Peter felt some relief, but after a few weeks, the panic attacks came back as intensively as previously. Again, he started thinking that he might have a real illness. His therapist tried some cognitive work on probabilities for different illnesses. Although Peter was open to the reasoning, his attacks did not cease. Peter's grandmother had died some months earlier; the therapist tried to help Peter become aware of feelings that had been evoked at the time. Peter talked about sadness and guilt over too rare visits, but the therapist did not feel that they really got hold of any strong emotions.

The therapist by and by realized that Peter's search for tools and her assistance in finding them had become a problem by itself. His desperateness was infectious; she felt as exasperated as he did. She talked with him about it. First, Peter did not understand and expressed frustration about this perspective on their mutual work. After a while, however, issues of success and failure, performance expectations, desire to have his suffering accepted came to the fore. He described situations where people had either belittled him for his problems or suggested simplified solutions. He felt like a failure. It was not difficult for the therapist to recognize similar feelings. After some more work on issues of vulnerability and the meaningfulness of challenges, Peter left therapy with less frequent anxiety attacks and a more humble view of life.

The therapy episode shows how the participants, inadvertently and with good intentions, end up in a locked situation that, when attended to, becomes material that can be used for mutual reflection. The material to work on is not what the patient brings to the therapy but the unfolding interaction between them (Benjamin, 1990).

An ethical perspective on two-person psychology

Realizing that the therapeutic relationship is co-created means that moral issues are mutual problems. The therapist's value system is always an aspect of the interaction. Active participation means that the therapist cannot hide in silence or anonymity. Should the patient make an abortion? Or break with his mother? Gazzaniga noted that "responsibility is a dimension of life that comes from social exchange, and social exchange requires more than one brain. When more than one brain interacts, a new set of rules comes into play, and new properties—such as personal responsibility—begin to emerge. The properties of responsibility are found in the space between brains, in the interactions between people" (2018, p. 232). Ethical issues are shared. Every breath will reveal the therapist. Therapeutic humility should bestow dignity to the patient and his challenges (Drozek, 2015; Shabad, 2001) and make the impossibility to remain outside ethical struggles evident (Rosen, 2012).

The two-person perspective has helped uncover the blindness in "institutionalized, normative abuse of power" (Hoffman, 2016, p. 95) in interventionist, medical models of psychotherapy. Professional ethics defined as rules and regulations by boards and organizations are important as baselines. However, in addition, as relational therapy presupposes engaged affective relating, ethical issues are part of the dialogue (Allen, 2016).

Construction and truth

Psychoanalytic treatment has always grappled with the issue of truth. Starting with the model that the patient should explore the historical and mental causes of symptoms, passing through the idea that the patient constructs his life narrative, psychoanalytic theory today is largely based on the perspective of truth as an ongoing process. Relational truth is provisional and open to revision, it does not lead to new and better understanding, it leads to new ways to understand (Hoffman, 1983, 1998; Mitchell, 1993; Stern, 1983). What the patient learns in therapy is a stance towards truth-seeking rather than truths. Truth is in the immediate emotional reality between analyst and patient, sometimes possible to be generalize to life (O'shaughnessy, 1994).

There needs to be a balance, however. Truth is also the necessary berthing to history in order not to slip over in pure fantasy (Blum, 2003). Although understanding life may be construed in various ways, facts cannot (Davies, 2018). The exploration of new perspectives, open-mindedness with regard to what happened and what happens (Renik, 1998), is in a continuous dialectic with objective reality.

One-person relational therapies

The focus on co-creation is the major addition of relational therapy to other contemporary dynamic therapy orientations. Both mentalizing-based and affect-focused therapies underline the importance of using the therapeutic relationship for understanding the patient's problems. But, in general, they retain the interventionist idea of the therapist as director of the treatment.

Several psychological methods are relational in the sense that they help the patient deal with their relationships, in the therapy relationship or outside. An evident example is family therapy where the relationships in the family are the main therapeutic concern. Another example is Interpersonal Therapy (IPT; Weissman, Markowitz, & Klerman, 2018), a treatment for psychiatric conditions like depression, anxiety syndromes, and eating disorders. It focuses on how the patient can deal with relationship problems that are related to his psychiatric problems. IPT is solution focused, it encourages the patient to find ways to handle conflicts or problems in his social network. Unlike relational therapy, the relationship between therapist and patient is not the focus of the therapeutic work (Markowitz, Milrod, Luyten, & Holmqvist, 2019). The therapy relationship is rather a secure base for dealing with other relational problems.

In some relational methods, the focus is on the actual therapeutic relationship. In schema therapy, recurring patterns in the patient's relational history are identified in the relationship between patient and therapist (Young, Klosko, & Weishaar, 2003). Another example is Functional Analytic Psychotherapy (FAP; Kohlenberg & Tsai, 1991) where the patient's behaviour in the session is used to detect problematic ways of relating outside therapy. FAP is a therapy in the Skinnerian tradition; the therapist's tools are based on operant conditioning. If the patient is excessively pleasing or submissive, the therapist may ignore such behaviour and reinforce more assertive behaviour.

In contrast to these methods, the therapist does not have a prerogative in understanding what happens in relational therapy. Not only the patient's relating behaviour, but the actual co-created interaction, is open for reflection.

Selves, spaces, and intersubjectivity

Do we have a core self? Or do we have different selves in different relational contexts? Perhaps the notion of a self is just a misuse of language? Questions about the continuity and coherence of the self are important in philosophy as well as in psychology (Mitchell, 1993). Some philosophers have argued that the notion of a self is a misconception, a reification of feelings of recollection or recurrence, but without any specific ontological platform that can with reason be called the self (Ryle, 1949; Wittgenstein, 1953). In ordinary speech, we can say "I promised myself" without implying that there is an agent experienced as myself. The reference is back to the person speaking but without really meaning that this self exists as a constant entity.

The idea of a core self is what we take for granted: I have the sense that I am the same person over time and situations. Although I can move between feelings states or mind sets, I remain the same person. Using a spatial metaphor, the self can with this perspective be likened to a building with different rooms. Although I can move between the rooms, it is still the same building. Thinking from this model, a person "owns" his self and his secrets, he is master in his mind. Some aspects may not even be apparent to the person, like a hidden "true self", but they are still parts of the core self (Winnicott, 1963).

Multiple selves

In the models of the mind that grew out of Klein's, Fairbairn's, and Bion's theories, the id was successively and in different ways transformed to parts of self-object constellations. Subjectivity was understood as moving from one mode of self-experience in a specific affective relationship with a specific kind of object representation to another self-object constellation, evoking behaviour in relationships that are congruent with the self-object representations. These models of multiple selves are temporal rather than spatial; the different selves appear in different contexts at different occasions. The multiple self is a self in process, similar to a music experience or the flow of a river (Mitchell, 1993; Rapaport, 1957).

Models of the mind serve pragmatic purposes. They are metaphorical ways to understand mental problems and the ways to work with them in therapy. The multiple self, or self-state, model implies that the mind can be seen as a combination of different subject positions or modes associated with expectations of relations with others. The doors can be tightly locked; the separate self-states can be strongly sequestered or rigidly held apart, dissociated. Restrictions in the fluidity between self-states may hamper fullness of experience, imagination, emotional depth, and capacity for intimacy. But when the individual functions optimally, the self-states are cohesive and mutually knowable (Bromberg, 2006; Stern, 2010). Bromberg suggested that mental health can be described as the capacity to "stand in the spaces between realities without losing any of them – the capacity to feel like one-self while being many" (Bromberg, 1993, p. 166).

An illustration:

The patient is in therapy for recurrent depressions. Last week, he made a serious suicide attempt and was brought to the emergency room. The therapist read about it in the shared medical record. When she meets him and asks about it, he admits but is hesitant to talk about it. It was just an impulse, he says. Since some time, he has a relationship with a woman whom he loves very much. He has not told her about his suicide attempt. When he is with her, he never thinks about suicide. He has, however, told his ex-wife about what happened. She knows that he has tried before; during their relationship, he several times threatened her to harm himself. At the next session, the patient, when questioned, admits that he has hundreds of pills saved for future suicide plans. His ex-wife has known this for a long time, but he has not told the therapist previously although they have talked thoroughly about his suicide thoughts. The therapist becomes angry and worried, and wonders what else she does not know.

In the coming sessions, they explore how the patient systematically but without conscious intents talks about, and stages, different aspects of himself in different relationship, partly based on his fantasies about how different persons would react to different pieces of information but also on what feels important in the different relationships.

Trauma and dissociated self-states

To live is to experience traumas (Kohut, 1984). Some persons experience more horrible events, threatful abuse, adverse relationships than others. Severe traumatic experiences are a common reason for getting therapy. The redirection of interest from traumas and dissociation to intrinsic motives and fantasies was the beginning of psychoanalysis proper (Howell, 2011). The relation between psychoanalysts and trauma-focused therapists and researchers has been complicated and marked by a "legacy of mistrust and misunderstanding" for a long time (Davies & Frawley, 1992). Since the divide between psychoanalysts and trauma researchers like Charcot and Janet in the 1890s, these traditions have developed without virtually any contact. Trauma therapists have continued to focus on integration of dissociated self-states as a treatment goal (Kluft, 1999). In this tradition, there is largely a consensus that treatment should proceed in stages. The patient needs to feel safe and stable in the therapeutic relationship before opening up to traumatic memories, and finally coming to a point where integration and reconciliation can take place (Briere, 1997; Nijenhuis et al., 2010).

An opening for understanding dissociative states caused by sexual and physical abuse among psychoanalysts was initiated when alternatives to the tripartite structural model of the mind were formulated, notably as multiple self-state models (Davies & Frawley, 1992; Mitchell, 1993). An effect of traumatic abuse, particularly from attachment persons, may be dissociation. It is too painful to take in the reality that the person who cares for you also wants to use and abuse you. The victim "obfuscates ... awareness of what is going on, because to see it clearly would threaten your ability to believe in those who are supposed to be caring for you ... it would threaten your attachment to your parents and as such, it would threaten your very survival" (Davies, 2019, p. 167). Instead, the victim puts away the experience in unformulated self-states, in oblivion.

Standard trauma treatments use a one-person perspective. Using a metaphor, the therapist is a savior standing on the shore, throwing out a rope or holding out a helping hand to the almost drowning patient (MacIntosh, 2015). With a two-person perspective, the therapist gets into the water, sometimes even losing her foothold. The integration of dissociated parts of the self is, in this model, a mutual process. Disavowed self-aspects, sometimes from both participants, contribute to mutual enactments (Chefetz & Bromberg, 2004). The trauma becomes visible as developments of fluid and complex multiple selves (Davies, 1999; Mitchell, 1993). Attempts to formulate them may evoke shame and even more dissociation. Often, the refuted self-states are enacted between therapist and patient. "As analysis progresses, the patient and analyst will live out the trauma that brought the patient to treatment" (Salberg, 2019, p. 638).

An illustration:

The patient's father was an alcoholic, his mother had a bipolar disorder. During several periods in his childhood, he had been in foster homes. In therapy, he felt a strong need to talk in detail about his painful childhood memories. The therapist listened carefully. But by and by, she started feeling that the patient repeated his stories in a somewhat compulsive way, requiring that she listen without commenting. The therapy was felt as idling. Finally, she tried to mention something about her feelings. The patient became hurt.

The next session, the patient came to a locked door; the therapist had forgotten their time. When the therapist realized that she had forgotten the time, she called the patient to apologize. The patient responded curtly. When they met, the therapist again apologized and asked how the patient felt about her mistake. He admitted that he was irritated but said that he had realized that the therapist has a lot to do and may easily become forgetful. The therapist felt that the pardon came too easily. Although remorseful, the therapist also felt a sting of irritation. The patient had gotten the upper hand and seemed to rejoice about it. The therapist thought she was in a predicament. It seemed insensitive to comment to the patient about his attitude although that was what she really would want to. The patient continued talking about his hardships in childhood. The therapist thought that he wanted to give her bad conscience: abandoned in childhood, abandoned by his therapist. Finally, she disclosed her thoughts. The patient started crying. At first, she felt a distance to his tears. Thinking about that, she felt shameful.

It struck her that she had foreclosed her thoughts about why she forgot the patient. She realized that leaving somebody out had a meaning in her own life. As an adult, she had been criticized by her sister for abandoning her as a child. She always thought her sister exaggerated but knew there was truth in it. Without saying anything about her life, she said to the patient that it had struck her that they had not talked about his ideas about why she forgot him. The patient looked sad and said that he realized that he could not be the most important person in her life. The therapist remembered that her sister used to say that no one was as important to her as she herself. Next time, she asked the patient to describe how it felt to be taken away from his family. When he did, she felt that she got tears in her eyes.

The illustration shows how split-off parts of the self may come to the fore in enactments where the therapist is caught in behaviour and feelings that seem incomprehensible outside the ongoing relationship. "The patient becomes stuck in a terrifying world of repetition where the relationship is assumed to be irreparably damaged ... The analyst is caught in a dissociated moment of their own and places the blame for the mess on the patient. It is only by wriggling out from under this oppressive fog of dissociation that something new, different, and surprising bursts open; a new co-constructed experience" (MacIntosh, 2015, p. 523).

Intersubjectivity

Intersubjectivity was introduced in the psychoanalytic literature by Stolorow (1978), a psychoanalyst in the Kohutian tradition. Stolorow and Atwood (1984) described intersubjectivity as the mutual influence of participants in relationships. No person can be understood in isolation, the self is always part of an intersubjective interplay, a system of reciprocal mutual influence (Orange, Atwood, & Stolorow, 1997). The relational context gives the frame, possibilities, and limits in all relationships. Within the frames, the participants form rules and positions dialectically. Modes of regulating affects and behaviour structure the interaction.

In contrast to this regulatory perspective, Benjamin (1990) argued that the key aspect of intersubjectivity is recognition. Using the Hegelian metaphor of master and slave, she described how intersubjectivity depends on recognition of the other's subjectivity and autonomy. The master can force the slave to show her respect, but genuinely felt respect presupposes that the master gives autonomy to the slave, implying the slave's right to deny her respect.

A milestone in the child's development is his recognition of the parent's own subjectivity (Benjamin, 2017). The child moves between the view that the mother can be dominated, and the insight that mother has her own will, her own subjectivity; sometimes she is happy, sometimes tired. Love cannot be forced; it can only be received. Recognition of the other's subjectivity is the measure of secure attachment.

Shared consciousness

Sterba (1934) suggested that a major goal in therapy is for the patient to identify with the therapist's observational ego. In relational therapy, this is described as mutual interest in the "relational unconscious". Researchers on the interaction between parent and child have formulated ideas about a relational (or dyadic) consciousness and a relational unconscious (Gerson, 2004; Tronick, 2003). These ideas have to a large extent developed from detailed studies of the interactions between parents and children (Brazelton et al., 1974; Stern, 1971; Trevarthen, 1974). Such studies led to the idea that psychological organization should not primarily be seen as a property of the individual but of the mutual system (Sander, 1977). "Age-appropriate forms of meaning ...

from one individual's state of consciousness are coordinated with the meanings of another's state of consciousness" (Tronick, 2003, p. 475).

The potential space

The shared potential space is a specific form of intersubjectivity. An illustration:

> In a theatre performance, one of the actors has a role where he plays a sadistic person. On the stage, he harasses his antagonist. As a spectator, I find it unpleasant and frightening. But I do not enter the stage to stop him. Gradually, the uncanny feeling grows that the actor enjoys being sadistic. When he says his lines, he is so aggressive that I sense that he shows his real feelings. I do not enter the stage in this situation either. But something happens with my experience. I lose the illusion, I become occupied by the concrete reality, by questions about the personality of the actor, the relationship between the two actors outside the stage. I may, to be sure, think that good actors have to use their own personality, their own experiences to make the play vital and engaging. Or, maybe an antisocial personality problem shown on the stage?

A defining characteristic of the play aspect of the experience is that the actors would never be asked if the performance is real or "just play" (Winnicott, 1971a). It takes place in an intermediate area, presenting another kind of truth than the factual. The playing child should never be asked "Did you conceive of this or was it presented to you from without?" (Winnicott, 1953, p. 239). Playing belongs to a special place, a transitional, potential space.

Novels and pieces of art are in the potential space, in borderland between pure fantasy and concrete reality. If the novel does not have any emotional contact with reality, it will lack vitality and meaningfulness, if it is only concrete reality, it becomes factual biography and does not invite the reader's creative fantasy. The potential space has one opening towards the inner mental life and one towards concrete reality. The teddy bear is concrete but takes its significance from the child's fantasy, engagement, and love.

In the past century, the cultural world started experimenting with the distinction between the concrete world and the potential space. When Duchamp exhibited his Bottle Rack in 1914, he challenged the limits of the potential world. Can a concrete, functional object take on the characteristics of an art piece? Something to play with, something that evokes fantasies? Theatre plays where the audience is invited to act on the stage and autofictional books and films are other challenges.

The potential space experience is usually not in focus for awareness although participants may become aware of it. The film illusion is something else than the documentary. Sometimes, the transition from the inner world through the potential space to reality comes gradually. You wake up from a dream with your partner at your side. In your dream, your partner betrayed you. You are still angry at him. He looks at you and you tell him what he did. You know very well it was a dream and you know that he has nothing to do with it. Or does he? You struggle with how to let go of the feeling of hurt or deception, how to let go the subjective imprint on the concrete world.

Potential space and psychotherapy

At its conception, transference was seen as a repetition of old experiences, as a template to put on new experiences. Today, transference and counter-transference are understood to emerge in the interaction, as potential new ways of relating based on previous experiences. The interaction moves in a dialectic between recurrent ways of constructing relationships and new ways of being in a relationship. The ongoing affective relational experience has a Janus faces, one turned towards memories, the other towards the future. The potential space is not only a place for co-constructing old experiences and expressing heretofore unformulated memories; it is also a room for "generative interventions" that make possible imagination of new possibilities (Cooney, 2018; Davies, 2018).

The third

In a novel, the story has a life of its own, like a third subject, in the intermediate area between the words written by the author and the reader's fantasy. When read, it is created in the reader's mind. But it does not belong to the reader, it cannot be directed by her. The concept "analytic third" attempts to capture such experiences in therapy. When two people meet, a relational atmosphere or culture may develop that is felt to have a life of its own that cannot be predicted or directed in advance (Ogden, 1994a, 2004). We create the relationship – and the relationship creates us. A close relationship begets a life of its own that we go along with. To call this inter-subjective experience "the third" plays with the idea that it is a separate subject. It suggests that the third affects the relationship between me and the other in a similar way as we as participants influence it. Illustrations may be to dance together or to joke together; the rhythm, the atmosphere takes over – and limits our interactional possibilities.

Benjamin (2004) made a distinction between two variants of the third: "the-one-in-the-third" and "the-third-in-the-one". The one-in-the-third denotes experiences like the rhythm between two dancing persons, the coordinated movements and sounds between a child and a parent. It is the pre-symbolic experience of recurrent patterns of mutual bodily and mental interaction.

The third-in-the-one, the symbolic or moral third, is the introduction of a third perspective in a relationship. It may be the marking a parent makes when she empathizes with the child, mirroring the pain and at the same time indicating that her sense of pain is not the same as the child's. The third in this sense may indicate that an experience is in the potential space. "We both know that what we are in now is not (only) the concrete reality". In many social contexts, paraphernalia are used to indicate that what happens takes place in a special, potential space. The stage, church liturgy, the therapy room. In the transference-countertransference situation, the participants know that their images and feelings exist in a special space. The fantasy of taking a beer together does not lead to the pub after the session (Benjamin, 2004).

The opposite of the observational third is collapse of reflection, loss of perspective. Relational moves are felt as necessary. The partners feel obliged to interact in certain ways, they cannot find the way out of constrained labyrinths. "Absence of thirdness is a corollary of the individual's inability to maintain a sense of potential space in their experience of themselves in the world" (Slavin, 2007b, p. 601). This way of experiencing has the quality of "brute reality" (Gentile, 2007), of "it is what it is" (Ogden, 1988).

Potential space and mentalizing

The potential space offers possibilities to explore the relationship with openness, uncertainty, and curiosity. In this regard, it has obvious similarities with mentalizing. Mentalizing also implies an openness for uncertainty, in the middle ground between cocksureness and lack of engagement. Potential space and mentalizing have grown from different theoretical and clinical traditions but both concepts can be used to describe an individual's curiosity about the world and about intersubjective experiences.

Mentalizing means to have a perspective on experiences that is neither self-evidentially certain ("psychic equivalence") nor only imagined ("pretend mode"; Allen, Fonagy, & Bateman, 2008). When mentalizing, experience is decoupled from absolute certainty about reality but anchored in it (Allen et al., 2008, p, 17). It is an "imaginative mental activity" (Fonagy, Gergely, & Target, 2007, p. 288).

According to Bram and Gabbard (2001), the two concepts are similar on four points: (1) they have their origin in the caregiver – child relationship, (2) they are used to describe variants of play with ideas and symbolic thoughts, (3) they may contribute to therapeutic change, and (4) they may be seen as therapeutic goals. In addition, both concepts capture states of *engaged uncertainty*. They are consequential for the participants' understanding of relational processes by allowing them to reside mentally in the borderland between convinced certainty and disengaged fantasy.

There are also a number of dissimilarities between the concepts (Bram & Gabbard, 2001):

a   Potential space is a broader concept than mentalizing; it also captures feelings of vitality in cultural experiences. Mentalizing is limited to expressions of mental functioning and their implications for mutual interaction.

b   Potential space is a conscious mental activity (although usually not at the centre of attention) whereas mentalizing may denote implicit and procedural knowing.

c   Mentalizing is (usually described as) an individual capacity whereas potential space is a way of experiencing relationships intersubjectively.

Mentalizing is an ability. It develops during childhood, based on the child's attachment security and capacity for perspective-taking. The capacity to mentalize changes over situations, but at least its explicit aspects are measurable as traits and can improve, for example, in mentalization-oriented therapies. It is meaningful to say that a person is more or less capable of mentalizing (Fonagy, 1999b); even self-rating scales have been created (Fonagy et al., 2016).

Potential space does not lend itself to empirical study in a quantitative sense. It would be a misconception to compare degrees of potential space. The potential space is "a frame of mind in which playing might take place" (Ogden, 1985, p. 139). Who can say if a person is in this frame of mind? Is it possible for the person himself to identify whether he is in the potential space? Or for an observer? Is it meaningful to say: "Now we are in a potential space"? Could anyone refute such a statement? The concept potential space is an experiential possibility that can be described but hardly measured.

Mentalizing, potential space, and mindfulness

In order to understand similarities and differences between mentalizing and potential space, it is instructive to compare them with still another concept: mindfulness. Mindfulness means a state of mind where the person attends to the content of his mind without evaluating what comes up. It is a natural state in humans that can be trained (MacDonald & Muran, 2020). In contrast to mentalizing, only the person herself can tell whether she is mindful. It would be odd to say that another person is mindful; you could say that he looks mindful or behaves in a mindful way. Mentalizing, on the other hand, is basically assessed by an observer.

Both mindfulness and mentalizing are individual states of mind, although mentalizing has been studied as a dyadic phenomenon (Möller, 2018). Potential space is a characteristic of the subject's experience of the outer world, whether it be a book or another person. Whereas both mentalizing and mindfulness can be trained, potential space is an emergent experience. It is possible to create conditions for potential space to emerge, but not to train being in this state.

Limits of potential space

Potential space offers possibilities but there are conditions that make this kind of experience impossible or hard to attain. Examples are patients who somatize their emotional suffering (Magnenat, 2016), and patients with psychotic tendencies who take their experiences for truth (Bion, 1962).

Another example where the use of potential space is complex is trauma work. In these therapies, the therapist may have the position of witness to the patient's traumas. The witness's position entails both a demand to explore and confirm the patient's experience and, at the same time, to offer a mental space for reflection.

In trauma therapy, the cousin of the potential space, the moral third position, can be used to underline lawfulness, a wish to repent and to put things right (Davies, 2018). It can be a "live third", a witness who can see and acknowledge what the unseeing "dead third" was blind to (Gerson, 2009). But this third subject can also open for reflection on more nuances in understanding traumatic experiences.

An illustration:

The patient recounts memories of repeated sexual abuse in her teens. The patient used to be in groups with adolescents who were known for abusive and violent behaviour. Some sexual encounters were outright rapes. The therapist asks for details, the patient is reluctant but describes them.

- So he actually forced you to ask him to penetrate you.
- I guess I provoked him. We were both drunk. We had done it before. I said no and tried to stop him; I think I cried. But when he did it, I didn't protest.
  The description evokes strong feelings in the therapist. She interprets the situation along her own reactions.
- I reckon you thought it was terrible. You were so young, and he didn't bother about you.
  This is validation of the experience but has a taint of psychic equivalence. In a pretend mode, the therapist might say.
- So you thought it was ok considering your previous experiences. I wonder whether you felt that you in some sense liked it.
  A teleological stance would be to focus on the activity.
- What did he actually do? Did he force you by violence or just by words?

These are all potentially reasonable interventions. In an attempt to invite to reflection, the therapist might ask the patient to describe what happened.

- I guess you might have felt a number of things in this situation. Sometimes persons are not aware of all of them. Would it be ok for you to tell me in detail what happened?
  The patient describes the rape, with the therapist asking for feelings at some places. The patient seems to be quite shameful about not having stopped the man. The therapist thinks that, although extremely

offensive, many persons may have had similar experiences. She decides to attempt some mentalizing.

- I understand that you were scared. What do you think the boy thought? Did he realize that?
- Some days afterwards, he called me and asked how I felt. It may sound strange, but I think he thought we both liked it. He became sad when I told him how I felt.

The patient, seemingly, tolerated reflection about the interaction. She could have become angry at the therapist and felt misunderstood. Then, they would have a possibility to reflect on fear of not being seen and believed, being abandoned with one's guilt and shame, feeling stupid. The line between invitation to reflection and re-traumatization is thin.

Recurrent patterns and emergent experiencing

The psychotherapeutic situation is a workshop. The work should lead to constructive living outside the workshop. In some methods, the focus is on teaching tools and techniques to be used outside the room, after the session. Mindfulness meditation and exposure techniques are trained in the session and used afterwards. Other methods target work on material that the patient brings to the session, like maladaptive thought patterns, dreams, narratives of problematic interpersonal situations. The task is for the therapist to recognize patterns in the material that the patient brings, to convey understanding and insight. An early metaphor for psychoanalytic work was to excavate remnants from the past. Loewald (1960) replaced this metaphor with the idea of a sculptor chipping away non-essentials, thus moving from detecting to creating. With all these perspectives, the material is brought to the session.

Transference work is a special case. The patient brings himself, his ongoing reactions to the therapy. The therapist attempts to transform them to material. She may help the patient discover that fantasies and feelings towards the therapist are in fact repetitions of recurrent relational patterns; transference templates (Freud, 1912b), attachment patterns (Bowlby, 1988), interpersonal cycles (Wachtel, Kruk, & McKinney, 2005), core relational conflicts (Luborsky & Crits-Christoph, 1990), cyclical maladaptive patterns (Levenson, 2017), schemas (Young et al., 2003), or reinforcement-based behavioural patterns (Tsai et al., 2009). The recurrent relational patterns are expressions of resistance to change. The patient "tries to change while staying the same" (Bromberg, 1998, p. 133). The therapeutic work is to detect, explore, and change dysfunctional patterns.

The scientific knowledge about recurrent patterns is solid (Albani et al., 1999). Attachment patterns, for instance, influence the way we interact throughout life, although they may change under specific circumstances (Luyten, 2015). Everyday experience corroborates the idea. A shy person is shy when she meets new people. But persons also change depending on whom they meet. The shyness may fade when she meets an accommodating and interested person. This is also what happens in the therapeutic relationship, for the patient as well as for the therapist. The patient who is self-confident in contacts with other people is self-confident with the therapist also. But the self-confidence may be shattered if the therapist challenges the patient's way of talking about his problems and his life. In the same way, the contact-creating therapist has her style with patients but can become silenced and quiet if the patient makes a confused or threatening impression.

Emergence

There are several reasons for questioning the usefulness of models based on the idea of interactive patterns recurring in the therapeutic relationship. On a pragmatic level, the model of the therapist as an authoritative interpreter of repetitive patterns in the patient's relationships is often unproductive. The collaborative curiosity that most therapy methods recommend may be hard to uphold if the therapist claims to have privileged knowledge about the mutual interaction.

The epistemological critique targets the untenable position that the therapist has an unobjectionable understanding of the ongoing relationship. If the interaction is created by both participants in a seamless way and knowledge about it construed mutually, how can the therapist know to what extent the interaction is based on previous experiences?

Humanistic therapies often skip historical exploration of the patient's reactions in therapy and focus on the usefulness of emerging interactional experiences for the future. The aim of therapy is to explore resources, to open for unseen potential. Relational therapy is, although not always acknowledged, inspired by such ideas.

Relational models of recurrent patterns

The dialectic between recurrent patterns and emergent experiences is central in relational theory. No one would deny the fact that persons tend to use old interactional patterns in new relationships. People have "a pervasive tendency to preserve the continuity, connections, familiarity of one's personal, interactional world" (Mitchell, 1988, p. 33). The essential question is what the dialogue about and the interaction around these discoveries lead to, how "co-creation of new interpersonal experience [may arise] out of the dust of more pathological reenactments" (Davies, 2016, p. 362).

In an attempt to reconcile the ideas of recurrency and emergency, Wachtel (2008) proposed to use Piaget's concepts of assimilation (including new information in old structures) and accommodation (changing structures based on new information). The question is how this is made in practice. If relational discoveries about emotional interplay and mutual fantasies emerge in the ongoing interaction, will they be assimilated to old patterns or used to create new?

Relational theory offers two kinds of answer. One is focused on skills and competencies like mentalizing, affect consciousness, and conflict resolution skills. "The emphasis in Brief Relational Therapy is on developing a generalizable skill of mindfulness rather than on gaining insight into and mastering a particular core theme" (Safran & Muran, 2000, s. 179). In the ongoing work on what the patient brings, the mutual efforts contribute to develop relational skills.

The other answer is about vitalizing experiences, decisive mutual events, moments of intensive and meaning-enhancing feelings. Emergent experiences do not copy previous patterns or experiences; they are new, but they speak with older events, they contradict them, or interpret them, or nuance them.

6   Problems, goals, procedures, and processes

In all therapies, distinctions can be made between the problem, the goal, the procedure to achieve the goal, and the actual change process. A cancer patient brings his problem, a tumour, to the physician. The aim may be to cure, or to increase life quality. The doctor uses a procedure, like surgery or prescription of cytostatic medication. These procedures hopefully bring about change by removing or reducing the tumour in mechanical or chemical ways. Whatever the specific problem or method, this pattern of problem → goal formulation → procedure → change process holds for treatments in general.

In psychological treatments, the patient may bring problems like lack of hope and vitality, anxiety reactions, a destructive lifestyle, problematic interpersonal situations, or unregulated feelings. Together, patient and therapist select among the troubles and define a goal, a focus (Summers & Barber, 2011). Using the therapeutic procedure, the therapist, in cooperation with the patient, tries to find interventions to apply on the material. Hopefully, the interventions activate change mechanisms like mentalizing, awareness and tolerance of affects, improved vitality, insight about disavowed representations. These mechanisms are assumed to change the problems the patient brought.

The problem in psychological therapies is that we seldom know whether the procedure really leads to the actual change mechanism. Looking at therapy from the perspective of the health care system, it is natural to ask for improvement in terms of reduction of diagnoses or symptoms. The evidence movement has supported such targets by publishing lists of evidence-based treatments for psychiatric syndromes (Chambless et al., 1996).

Although psychotherapy often has had an ambivalent position in relation to the goals of medical psychiatry, psychoanalysis was for decades closely allied with the medical perspective. The first psychoanalysts were physicians; in the United States, only physicians were allowed as members of the American Psychoanalytic Society until a few decades ago. Psychoanalytic theories have strongly contributed to the psychiatric diagnostic systems (Kernberg, 2002).

A purely psychological perspective on psychotherapy was first developed by behavioural therapists (Haynes & O'Brien, 1990). Successively during

DOI: 10.4324/9781003026914-6

many years, however, the critique against the medicalization of psychotherapy has grown also among psychoanalysts. Interpersonal and relational psychoanalysis played a decisive role in this development (Hoffman, 2009a; Hofmann & Hayes, 2019; Johnstone & Boyle, 2017).

Problems and material

Persons who seek psychotherapy are often not certain about the nature of their suffering or the goals they want to attain. They may feel bad, they may be depressed or anxious, uncertain about themselves and their relationships. The initial task in therapy is often to make some formulation about the problems and what should be dealt with in therapy.

In mental health care, the patient's emotional and existential suffering and problems are transformed to treatable problems. Sometimes, the framing is easy; the snake phobia should be overcome. But often, a process of inclusion and exclusion, a negotiation with the patient, has to take place. Emphasis is put on some aspects of the problem; other aspects are toned down. The therapist's treatment model is used to define the material.

In public health services, the problems that the patient brings usually become framed as diagnoses. When a diagnostic syndrome has been defined, treatment protocols may be applied. This model has in recent decades become predominant in many countries, but both behavioural and relational authors have sharply criticized this medical way of understanding psychological problems (Hoffman, 2009a; Hofmann & Hayes, 2019).

In talking therapies, the material to be worked on is usually brought to the session by the patient's descriptions of daily-life experiences: interactional episodes, thoughts, feelings, problematic behaviour. In psychoanalysis, in addition to stories and fantasies brought to the session, feelings and thoughts about the therapist are used as material. This material is thus not tied to problems that make the patient seek therapy initially. It would be odd if a patient started therapy in order to talk about his feelings about the therapist. The transference emerges in the therapeutic interaction. However, transference is understood as emanating from the patient's life history, as an expression of memories of previous interactions that become activated in the therapeutic relationship. As a therapeutic material, it is understood as reflecting interactional problems outside the therapeutic relationship.

In relational therapy, material that emerge in the ongoing mutual interaction is emphasized. The patient does not bring it, it evolves in the therapeutic relationship. The material is "enactments and reenactments in the intersubjective field" (Davies, 2018, p. 654). Although coloured by the life histories of both patient and therapist, the material emerges in the interaction. The material is created in the therapeutic interaction. "[The therapist's] material is an ever-shifting experiential context, the most powerful element of which first reaches him perceptually, not cognitively, because it is being enacted while other things are being spoken" (Bromberg, 2012a, p. 6). Thus, the focus of the work, the material to be worked on, depends on the sensitivity and creativity of both therapist and patient.

How to create relational material

Most therapists adhere to the simple rule to think first and speak afterwards, in contrast to everyday conversations, when people may talk without always knowing where it will end up. Therapeutic cautiousness is a good rule, in general. In relational therapy, however, there are good arguments for being more spontaneous than is usual in psychotherapy. If the therapist wants to contribute to the interaction, she has to interact. The therapist needs to play the game that emerges before commenting on it. Giving advice and suggestions, for instance, may sometimes be helpful. Not always for the wisdom of the recommendations but for the vitality of the conversation. If the therapist does not allow for some spontaneity and relational courage, she will never stumble, she will not create the interactional hassles that may become material for reflection (Hoffman, 1998).

The point in creating conditions for the emergence of a genuine relationship is not the activity per se. Often, silence is warranted. The approach is to become engaged, to be present, and at the same time put the ear to the ground in order to be attentive to under-meanings, hints, cues. Engagement may entail curiosity but also confrontation, even critique (Cooper, 2008; Hoffman, 1996).

An example:

- Last time you said you would try not to drink every night. It doesn't seem you've followed the plan. Why is that?
- It's not easy to get rid of old habits, especially as my wife takes a glass every night.
- I think it's important that you really try. If you don't, you will feel you've failed and we will both become disappointed.
- Easy for you to say.
- If we are going to get anywhere, you have to make an effort.

This dialogue may sound much too pushy for a psychodynamic therapist. It does not in any way open for the patient to reflect on his motives. But if there are good reasons at this particular stage in the interaction for the therapist to insist, this may be what the patient expects as a reaction to his drinking.

The conversation can proceed in different ways. Here is one:

- Everyone tells me I have to pull myself together. I feel ashamed of course when I drink.
- So you don't think I have much more to offer than others?

- Well you're more blunt when you tell me to stop.
- I guess both of us really want to understand why you are doing this?
- Yes, that's probably why I'm here.
- I was quite pushy of course and… well, what did you feel about that?
- I felt ashamed, I always do.
- So we end up with something, you and me. You promise to try and then you come back and … you didn't succeed. I get disappointed and frustrated and start to rebuke you. And you feel even more ashamed. It's like a trap that both you and I end up in. For me, it's as if I have a need to urge you at the same time as I feel queer doing it.

There could be other ways for the dialogue. The patient could have become angry with the therapist and the therapist had become defensive. Or the therapist could have come up with ideas about how the patient and his wife could behave so that the temptation would not be so great. In whatever way the conversation continues, the therapist's active engagement eventually leads to complications that create opportunities for both patient and therapist to reflect on what happens between them.

The dialogue illustrates that the material is created from the therapist's "overarching attunement … to his contextualized perceptual experience … an ever-changing field that is shaped by a felt disjunction between what is being enacted and what is being said" (Bromberg, 2012b, p. 283). Does this differ from the "evenly hovering attention" that Freud recommended (Freud, 1912a)? It does, and the difference is the therapist's active involvement in the interaction, and awareness of her personal contribution to both the actual interaction and how it is perceived and understood. The therapist does not only register her reactions; they are part of the material.

The idea to become part of the material by the focus on the ongoing interaction may for many therapists be felt as uncomfortable. This perspective opens for scrutiny of deliberate or unwitting disclosure of the therapist's person. The argument for this approach is that genetic interpretations ("doesn't our interaction resemble the way you used to interact with your mother?") or proposals to talk about affect-laden situations outside therapy are often expressions of therapist avoidance against uncomfortable feelings in the ongoing interaction. The dialogue above might have ended up in the patient's critic of the therapist's manner to be self-righteous, and she might have felt exposed on this point. That is also material.

Therapy goals

In traditional psychoanalysis, the goal of understanding repressed memories and fantasies, and the processes that uphold such repression was soon complemented by descriptions of development of mental capacities like the ability to embrace and tolerate the complexities of mental life, exemplified by the attainment of the depressive position (Etchegoyen, 1991), and the ability to accept ownership of dissociated parts of the self. Other definitions focus on the search for a true self, and transmuting internalizations leading to confirmation of the self (Kohut, 1984). Sterba (1934) argued that the goal was for the patient to identify with the therapist's observing ego. This has also been described as an ability to self-analyze, to create a psychoanalytic mind (Busch, 2014; Falkenström, 2007). Basic to these definitions is the idea that a person without ability to tolerate and be mindful about painful aspects of his mental world is a victim of repetition of patterns instead of being able to reflect on them.

In the relational literature, goal descriptions may sound like this: "[patients] …want to feel more satisfaction and less distress in their lives" (Renik, 2007, p. 1547), "changes in a patient's sense of self and ways of being in the world" (Hoffman, 2016, p. 93) or "ability to cope successfully with challenges, to develop, and to find a meaningful direction for their lives as long as it helps them understand and organize their self-experience in new, more operational, and harmonious ways" (Yerushalmi, 2018, p. 229). Relational therapy focuses on "more fundamental yet elusive issues, like the quality of being" (Black, 2003, p. 633). Ghent (1989, p. 207) made a list of potential goals:

- A need for protection of the self as well as all that is meaningful to it, including one's own body and the integrity of meaningful others.
- A need for a feeling of self-worth, dignity, self-esteem.
- A need for the expansion of awareness (and "aliveness"); for "knowing" as distinct from knowledge, the absence of which leads to feelings of "deadness".
- A need for inner integration of the self; the yearning to surrender "false self"; the quest for wholeness and unity, "centredness".
- A need for meaning, significance, and coherence.
- A need for growth, that is, the integration of new function, in distinction to the execution of already integrated function.

Although such goals may be understandable in a poetic sense, and certainly by many suffering persons, it is not the cup of tea for health authorities. The tension between relational goals and symptom reduction could be more vigorous and courageous than it is.

Implicit relational knowing

For many therapists, skills training is associated with behavioural therapies. In such therapies, training is usually deliberate and systematic. There are some examples of dynamic therapies that have as explicit objective the development of a skill, although usually less specific than in behavioural therapies. Mentalizing-oriented therapies and affect-focused therapies are examples of this. The Boston CPSG (2018) describes the goal of relational treatment as a "catalyzing of new capacities as patient and analyst move through the patient's most troubling vulnerabilities in increasingly fluent and flexible ways". Such a new or improved capacity may be mentalizing, a natural consequence of dialogs focused on mutual curiosity. To improve the patient's ability to be aware of, modulate, and express an ample range of feelings (Jurist, 2018; Lear, 2003; Shedler, 2010) is another expected effect of the relational focus.

Tolerance of uncertainty

One goal in relational therapy is tolerance for uncertainty. To be able to handle uncertainty has been underscored as a basic human capacity by many authors. "Ambiguity is of the essence of human existence. ... there is in human existence a principle of indeterminacy, ... it does not stem from some imperfection of our knowledge ... Existence is indeterminate in itself, by reason of its fundamental structure" (Merleau-Ponty, 1962, p. 169). Tolerance of uncertainty is the opposite of enactments; it is the essence of the potential space experience. The goal is multiplicity, plurality, it is to avoid closure of paradoxes (Pizer, 1998).

A tolerance for ambiguity and uncertainty as opposed to the more uni-directional, linear acquisition of specific, finite, objectively derived insight. (Davies, 2018, p. 660).

Ability to lead a meaningful life, to create vital relationships

The goals of many patients who start therapy are existential. They want to create more vital relationships, to find more meaning in life, to come to grips with one's life history, to develop one's potential, to explore dreams for the future. Such needs are often combined with wishes to get rid of anxiety, depression, or obsessive thoughts; symptom alleviation is often tied to changes in one's life situation. Patients do not usually seek therapeutic treatment just for symptoms but rather for lack of meaningfulness and life direction. Change may imply new ways of relating to others, new ways of looking upon oneself. Mitchell (1993) argued that the main goal for relational treatment is for the patient to regain or find his *authenticity*.

The idea of authenticity as a significant aspect of a person's ways of being or even a virtue has roots back to the 16th and 17th centuries (Safran, 2017). The reformation of the church underlined the demand for individual responsibility; the capitalist development also emphasized that the individual has her fate in her hands. The romantic movement in literature and art during the late 18th century focused on the expressiveness of the individual, her right and need to find her own ways. Existentialist authors like Kierkegaard, Heidegger, and Sartre elaborated on the struggles of contemporary man to find himself, his true, authentic self. Binswanger, a German psychiatrist, was the first to introduce authenticity as a concept in psychoanalysis. But not until the relational turn, concepts such as genu-ineness and authenticity became important as treatment goals among psy-choanalytic writers (Safran, 2017).

Procedures

In many therapy schools these days, procedures are called tools. In everyday talk, a tool produces a certain effect through a certain activity. A rake has teeth that tear up weeds. Mindfulness meditation and list writing are tools for patients with fatigue or ADHD. Such techniques can be taught by therapists, but also acquired as self-help.

The causal chain between problem, goal, procedure, and process may seem obvious with these methods. However, the scientific knowledge about why a particular activity leads to change in psychotherapy is limited (Cuijpers et al., 2019; Kazdin, 2005). Interestingly, Saul Rosenzweig, the author credited with the formulation of the common factors idea, already in 1936 noted that "besides the intentionally utilized methods and their con-sciously held theoretical foundations there are inevitably certain un-recognized factors in any therapeutic situation – factors that may be even more important than those being purposely employed" (p. 412).

In solution-focused treatments, it is often the patient who is taught and uses the tool. In relational therapy, the therapist uses the "tool". Not seldom, the patient may feel bewildered about the therapist's use of the procedure, especially as it may be unclear in what way the procedures lead to the therapeutic aim.

An example is work with alliance ruptures. In all therapy methods, there are ruptures and hassles in the therapeutic relationship. Hopefully, the therapist becomes aware of them and attempts to engage the patient in a collaborative attempt to understand what happens, and, if necessary, modify or redirect the work. Most therapists would argue that the alliance is im-portant as a carrier for the method. But the method is usually something else, like exposure or interpretation of unconscious intentions.

With a relational perspective, attendance to ruptures and mutual reflec-tion on them is an intervention, a procedure, that may lead to change. However, in the moment when rupture work is made, it is the ethos of re-lational therapy that is the motivator: to be curious about the interplay, engaged, genuine, and earnest. It may seem odd if the therapist, on such moments, deliberately thinks that by handling a difficult situation, she is using a method with the intent to improve the patient's mentalizing. It can certainly happen, but the situation illustrates the half-planned, half spon-taneous nature of relational therapy.

As the therapist actively contributes to the interaction, the distinction between material and procedure may seem unclear in relational therapy. Therapist self-disclosure, for instance, is often a spontaneous comment about the ongoing dialog. But it can also be a way of stepping out of an enactment to create a point of reflection about the interaction (Aron, 2006), in that sense being a therapeutic procedure. Is it, then, material to be understood or a procedure applied to the interaction?

Bromberg (2012b) argued that the relational turn implies three important changes from a traditional psychoanalytic stance: a focus on context rather than content, a focus on affect rather than cognition, and a decreased interest in technique (p. 283).

What then is the relational procedure? A typical description is: "our practice of psychoanalysis becomes more emotionally authentic, more spontaneous and inventive, more compassionate and liberating to both our patients and ourselves" (Benjamin, 2004, p. 42). Another description is that the therapist's stance is "personal attunement and validation" (Hoffman, 2016, p. 91). According to Bromberg (2012a), the therapeutic action is "a self/other negotiation that takes place between and within analyst and patient at the interface of dissociation and the capacity to hold internal conflict. It is a nonlinear process that endows both their relationship and their individual self-states with an ever-evolving experience of wholeness that is the primary source of healing and growth". Again, these are catching descriptions but hard to teach.

The relational procedures are approaches and stances rather than techniques. The focus is to become aware of, communicate about, and reflect on enactments that emerge in the therapeutic relationship. As noted earlier, the precondition is that the interaction allows for the kind of complications to develop that naturally arise when two persons genuinely strive to come to grips with complicated issues. "The interaction doesn't reek of therapeutic purposes at every moment. In fact, there are more times, more interludes, when the conversation sounds like one that might occur in ordinary social life" (Hoffman, 2009b, p. 624).

The rhythm in relational therapy is to move from focused discussions about problems that the patient brings to therapy to attention to complications that arise in the therapeutic interplay and reflections on it. When the focus moves to the therapeutic relationship, the dialogue is often called negotiation. Negotiation may sound like rational deliberations around sound arguments. Nothing could be further from the relational use of the concept. Negotiating is stumbling into unforeseen dilemmas and, through attending to dissonances and attempted restructuring, finding new places to get lost in.

Theoretically, negotiation may mean that "dissociated" states become recognized by the other (Benjamin, 2007), that the subject can "hold the other's mind in her mind" (Fonagy et al., 2002). The procedure has been called "state-sharing" of the right brain hemispheres (Schore, 2003), pointing to its emotional rather than intellectual aspect. In this process, the "relational unconscious", the thirdness, the experience of something more than the participants' individual contributions, opens for integration of warded-off or never formulated self-states (Stern, 2010). The decisive step is the recognition of felt but unthinkable, or at least unthought, intersubjective experiences. The therapist must be prepared to "enter into an intense relationship and to retain his function of putting experience in words" (Rosenfeld, 1987, p. 160). The therapist's task is to try to find multiple meanings, to recognize the patient's subjectivity and to appreciate the patient's recognition of the therapist's subjectivity.

Moving along and focusing

The traditional psychoanalytic stance of letting the transference material evolve in the ongoing interaction has been complemented by focused approaches in time-limited dynamic therapies. In Chapter 1, time in psychological change processes was discussed. It is a challenging issue whether the relational procedure is useful in shorter treatments. Is it meaningful to speed up the development of deep relationships? Is it meaningful to "play psychoanalysis" in 10 or 15 sessions (Sandell et al., 2000)? Is speed dating possible in therapy? One thing is to have an active therapist, quite another to create a viable relational process in a therapy that focuses on symptom improvement.

The creative moment

One aspect of relational procedures is that they need to be intuitive, "artistic". Moments of meeting, for instance, "must be seized if one is going to change his destiny, and if it is not seized, one's destiny will be changed anyway for not having seized it" (BCPSG, 2010, p. 42; Stern et al., 1998). In these moments, past and future may blend and enrich each other. "kairos, the spontaneous linking of past and present, in both directions, is the ideal of the mind's functioning" (Stern, 2017, p. 503). In these moments of enhanced vitality, meaningfulness, and "realness" (Mitchell, 1993), the authenticity of the therapist is probably a key factor (Duarte et al., 2020; Safran, 2017).

Davies (2018) described "generative interventions", interpretations that aim to change the perspective for the patient, open up new and heretofore unthought mental rooms. Generative interventions turn the eyes towards the current, ongoing creation of meaning. The goal is not to find out what *is*, but to create what *never has been* (Summers, 2016). The therapeutic relationship creates new forms of relating, new self-relations (Benjamin, 1995; Stern, 1997; Winnicott, 1971b). The creative interplay in the dyad is a possibility for patient and therapist to develop new relational forms and patterns (Harris et al., 2020).

Surrender

A specific form of procedure is surrender. Surrender means to let go, to give up, to accept (Ghent, 1990). Both patient and therapist may surrender to new ways of relating, to dependence and reliance on others. In the relational tradition, surrender was introduced and explicated by Ghent (1990). It is to believe in the therapeutic process, the non-directive flow. When other therapy models advocate goal-directedness, active recommendations, the relational model is to rely on the engaged interaction (Safran, 1999). This approach has its special value in processes that get stuck, in times of hopelessness and resignation. Instead of avoiding such states by introducing various solution suggestions, interpretations, and advice, the patient may need a therapist who stays with him in the dark night of the soul.

Curiosity

Psychotherapists always need to struggle against their preconceived ideas. Psychoanalytic theory is replete with models for understanding the patient's material. This is not unique for therapists who are allegiant to interpretative models; all therapists have ideas about how to understand what they hear, based on their unique experiences. The challenge is to combine set patterns with openness for new impressions. Stern (1997) suggested that the therapist use "dialogic epistemology" (Gadamer, 1975), implying that the therapist discloses, wittingly or not, her ideas about how to understand the patient, with as much of openness as possible about both her own and the patient's perspective. Instead of feigning open curiosity, a better way is to be open about the frames in the therapist's mind.

Technique and person

When asked whether research findings were helpful in his clinical practice, the legendary clinical researcher Paul Meehl answered: "Not at all!" (Goldfried, 2010). In a similar vein, technique in any formal sense is often dismissed by relational authors. Technique is the spontaneous relationship. "When I am with a patient, my self-experience is so highly organized through the relationship that being an analyst feels like being myself. Since I do not experience myself as doing analysis, any more than I experience myself as doing any relationship, the concept of technique does not enhance my understanding of what shapes the self I bring to an analytic relationship" (Bromberg, 2012a, p. 14).

However, the relationship is special. It is framed by the therapeutic task. There is spontaneity, but there is also a ritual (Hoffman, 1996). The ritual may differ between therapists, depending on training and personality. Given the specific tenets of relational theory, for example, the view that each patient, each therapist, and each therapy is unique and that mutual enactments alter the therapeutic needs continuously, it is hard to define overarching technical rules. "[the therapist] can no longer say with any certainty what he is actually doing, nor can he know why he is doing what he is trying to do" (Tublin, 2018, p. 73). Attempts to chisel out technique from person are elusive in relational therapy.

The therapist's contribution

One reason for Freud (1912b) to recommend the therapist to use "evenly hovering attention" was to ensure that the therapist would not become prejudiced in her attempts to understand the meaning in what the patient said. However, as Pine (1988) noted, it is impossible not to be influenced by preconceived ideas and concepts. Human listening is inherently meaning finding. It is basic to human nature to try to understand patterns in her perceptions, to categorize experiences and to put them in contexts that are familiar. No one would expect a Kleinian to find anything else than Kleinian meanings in her patients' associations. One thing is to strive to be non-evaluative, another is to succeed. The practice of psychoanalysis has always been hermeneutical (Allen, 2016), meaning that clinical models have decided which understanding is possible.

Understanding is subjective and situational. Another therapist, or the same therapist on another occasion, might contribute to another construal of the interaction (Hoffman, 2016). The intervention is not to solve riddles, it is to move between occasional understanding and renewed puzzlement, and to tolerate the uncertainty that the continuous therapeutic process begets. Ghent (1989) wrote that relational therapy "ultimately [is] a belief system that the analyst lives and works by ... [it] makes a very significant difference as to how one hears, what one hears, how one assembles what is heard" (p. 170).

Provided that mutual enactments are the key material in relational treatment, the therapist often does not know in what direction to go, she may feel confused and bewildered (Hoffman, 2009b). The dialogue between patient and therapist may seem inexact, unpredictable, and discontinuous. The therapist's position is radical uncertainty with regard to the significance of the patient's as well as her own participation (Stern, 2015). If the therapist thinks she knows, she is not in touch with the patient's real situation or the significant aspects of their interaction. The task is not to find the obvious, the task is to find the non-understandable, to become aware of the unfelt.

The intervention and the response

In some therapies, the influence of the intervention on the patient's response is assessed immediately. Exposure to frightening stimuli is like the knife and the tumour. Likewise, in dynamic therapy, the interpretation of a dream is a clear-cut intervention. The effects of the intervention can be observed and assessed, although the understanding of the response may be complex. In relational therapy, the response to interventions is difficult to assess in a straightforward way. Although some research and theoretical models suggest that patients may react immediately on relational experiences in the session (Falkenström, Ekeblad & Holmqvist, 2016; Falkenström & Holmqvist, 2021; Stern, 2004a, 2004b; Zilcha-Mano, 2019), it is more reasonable to think that the effects of the therapeutic work grow successively.

Processes of change

In the scientific literature, there are many proposals and little knowledge about the actual processes of change in psychotherapy (Kazdin, 2009). Cuijpers and co-writers recently remarked: "It is as if we have been in the pilot phase of research for five decades without being able to dig deeper if the aim of psychotherapy research is to understand how change comes about" (2019, p. 224). Therapists, unfortunately, often mix up procedure with process (Hofmann & Hayes, 2019; Kazdin, 2005); they, naturally, think that their interventions produce the change. In psychoanalysis, interpretations are often seen as the prime change agent (Messer & McWilliams, 2007; Sandler, Dare & Holder, 1973). Although a few empirical studies support the idea of insight as a factor leading to change (Johansson et al., 2010; Koelen et al., 2012), it is probable that change comes from many sources. In this section, relational hypotheses about change mechanisms are presented.

Reparation of relational expectations

Psychological change can be seen as relearning, reparation, or correction of old patterns or traumas in order to develop more constructive and creative ways to deal with relations and situations. Many authors suggest that experiences in therapy may function as reparation or compensation for previous dysfunctional relational experiences and expectations. Alexander and French (1946), partly basing their model on Ferenczi's (1933) ideas, coined the concept corrective emotional experience, meaning deliberate interventions to change dysfunctional patient expectations. More recent examples of reparative models are theories about cyclical interpersonal patterns (Wachtel, 2014) and plan formulations (Weiss, Sampson, & Mt Zion Psychotherapy Research Group, 1986).

The idea of therapy as a compensatory relational experience has evoked interest not only in psychoanalytic therapies (Castonguay & Hill, 2012). In relational theory, several different strands of thought about the therapeutic potential of reparative experiences have been formulated. One is the tradition from interpersonal psychoanalysis implying that mutual enactments in the ongoing therapeutic interplay is a pivot point for emotional change (Benjamin, 1996; Kiesler, 1986; Weiss et al., 1986). Already Sullivan wrote about "the drive toward mental health" (1953, p. 100); Winnicott assumed a "tendency towards growth …[in order to counteract] … mental illness as a hold up in development" (1989, p. 194). In this theoretical tradition, the interaction in therapy is a way to unlock the patient's urge to become mentally sane (Searles, 1975).

Another tradition comes from Ferenczi, suggesting that the therapist may compensate for parental neglect, for relational traumatic experiences. Balint (1968) suggested that the patient needs to come under the skin of the therapist in order to repair the "basic fault", unsettling both therapist and the mutual work. In this perspective, the therapist not only detects and explores enacted dysfunctional patterns; she becomes part of them in a "flow of enactive engagement" (Grossmark, 2012). Change, in this model, is brought about by the therapist's "attuned recognition" of the shared enactment (Salberg, 2019, p. 638). The idea of the therapist as a "bonus parent" has been advanced not only in psychoanalytic therapies. In schema therapy, for instance, "limited reparenting" is suggested as a therapist approach leading to fulfillment of unmet emotional needs (Young et al., 2003). The relational colour of this idea is the degree of emotional involvement in the therapist.

Vitalizing experiences

Intensive, affectively charged experiences may radically change a person's way of experiencing himself and his relationships. These moments, sometimes called moments of meeting or dyadic expansion of consciousness (Tronick, 1998, 2001), imply heightened affective interaction between patient and therapist (Beebe & Lachmann, 1994, 2020). Reciprocal emotional exchanges are thought to act as self-organizing processes in the dyadic system. The result may be an expansion of both partner's states of consciousness. The idea connects to Cooney's (2018) expression "vitalizing enactments" for moments when embryonic, underdeveloped affects and capacities can be potentiated. It is thus a view of enactment as progressive and creative. "In vitalizing enactment, the action is in seizing the moment and creating something new" (p. 343).

The discussion of future focusing in relational approaches, offering the patient (and therapist) vitalizing, enlivening hope is lively (Aron & Atlas, 2015; Davies, 2018; Director, 2016; Grossmark, 2012). Cooney (2018) for instance, makes a distinction between "seizing the moment and creating something new" in contrast to Aron's and Atlas' (2015) idea about "rehearsing future outcomes" and Davies' "generative interpretations". Director (2016) suggests that patients who have suffered emotional neglect may need the therapist as a "catalyst", a person who initiates development (Director, 2016). Several researchers have pointed to the importance of aligning with the patient's future directions in psychotherapy, to align with his directionality (Cooper, 2019; Oddli et al., 2021).

Attention to subtleties

A common idea is that attention to subconscious feelings, fantasies, and thoughts that have not reached the surface of consciousness may be a change mechanism in psychotherapy. In an ongoing interaction they may become conscious, sometimes with pain, sometimes evoking curiosity or fascination. The ability to become aware of nuances and subtleties in relationships has attracted interest from many authors. Gendlin (1996) described the "felt sense", meaning implicit body sensations, that may become translated to conscious experiences through a process that Gendlin called focusing. Bollas called a similar phenomenon the "unthought known" (Bollas, 1987), Schacter named it "procedural memories" (Schacter, 1996), Stern (1997) "unformulated experience", and Ogden (2001) as the "frontier of dreaming". These are experiences that are felt as insights and discoveries once they come in attention focus.

Such expansion of consciousness can take place without contact with someone else, but the relational idea is that it develops in affect-laden therapeutic interactions.

Implicit relational skills

Implicit relational knowing, to get a feeling for affective attunement, for subtle nuances in the interaction, is a vital aspect of human interaction (Boston CPSG, 2010). Such procedural competence usually remains out of conscious awareness. It is the competence to know when to talk and when to listen, when to laugh and when to be serious, how to know what to do when things go wrong, and how to know when and how to become intimate and confidential and when to keep an emotional distance (Lyons-Ruth, 1999). It is like riding a bike. The competence is learnt in childhood, it can be trained. But it is hard to explain verbally. Aron suggested that the Kleinian concept "unconscious phantasy" in fact expresses implicit procedural rules that remain unformulated phantasies until they are formulated with words in therapy (Aron, 2014, p. 343). Particularly the Boston CPSG has argued for this as the basic mechanism of change in therapy, as a process that takes place outside the awareness of patient and therapist.

Increased authenticity

To meet the therapist in an authentic and genuine way has been thought to be curative since Rogers. Often, authenticity is expressed by the therapist's improvisations and spontaneity. To break conventional or accepted therapeutic rules, "throwing away the book" (Hoffman, 1998), improvise (Knoblauch, 2000; Ringstrom, 2001) has at times become the rule in relational therapy.

An apparent problem with this idea is that it may open for the therapist's narcissism (Lunbeck, 2014). Ringstrom (2007) emphasized the ethical aspect of improvisation and the need to combine it with consideration of the patient's needs. Similarly, Stern (2004a) emphasized that the authentic response in the now moment must be intersubjectively fitting.

Authenticity needs a moral, it requires a struggle with one's systems of values and views of the human condition (Ringstrom, 2007; Taylor, 1992). An important aspect of authenticity is thus to *stand for something* (Calhoun, 1995). Going back to Rousseau, Grant (1997) pointed to goodness as a virtue in therapy. It is not only a matter of finding oneself; the question is about finding oneself as a person who has his own core of meaning and values. In the process of struggling for what one stands for, a sense of vitality and intense feeling may emerge. The therapist in this perspective has an apparent significance as a person, not only with personal traits and habits, but as a person of ethical principles.

Davies (2016) argued that there are several reasons to be sceptical about improvising in therapy as the main means to change. One is that if the interplay between therapist and patient is not made explicit the patient will continue seeing it with his old eyes. It is in the conscious reflection that the patient (and the therapist) become aware of new perspectives. Another reason is that the therapist may overestimate her ability not to be drawn into the patient's interactional patterns, into "relational projective identification" (Davies, 2016), for instance, by allowing and supporting idealization of herself. Finally, the best way to help the patient translate new relational experiences in the therapeutic relationship to relationships outside therapy is by making him or her visible in the therapeutic verbal dialogue. "The most important differentiation of the mind's contents is between subjectivity that can be used in the creation of authentic living and subjectivity that cannot be used in that way" (Stern, 2017, p. 503). The contrast to ideas in, for instance, the Boston CPSG about implicit processes that produce change without ever becoming conscious is obvious.

Opening closed rooms

Building on the idea that emotional problems are caused by split-off self-states, a prominent idea in relational therapy is that the patient changes when he can regain or even for the first time find new self-states, new openings in his mind, to give words to dissociated experiences (Bromberg, 2006). Bromberg (2012a) argues that the principle in all dynamic treatments is the development of intersubjectivity in areas of the mind that are captured by dissociative mental structures (p. 11).

Winnicott (1971b) and others (McDougall, 1993) have used the metaphor that the mother's unconscious is the child's first contact with reality. The implication is that the parent's untold wishes and feelings are more important than what he or she says openly. This metaphor opens for both the introjection of both healthy and destructive aspects of the parent's unconscious. The greater the gap between untold and told, the more of the child's experience becomes unformulated, in a split-off self-state (Davies, 2019).

In therapy, split-off parts of the patient (and therapist) may become visible as enactments. When the patient and therapist become aware of them, the patient will be recognized by the therapist (McKay, 2019). And the patient is not only is recognized; he also recognizes the therapist and can see her as a separate person (Davies, 2018).

Coda

The description of problems, goals, procedures, processes will be illustrated by two therapies with patients with similar symptoms. Both could probably have been treated with established methods for borderline patients like DBT and MBT.

Anne

Anne is 22. She has cut herself since she was 15. When her anxiety and despair are overwhelming, the pain from cutting relieves her anxiety. In therapy, she wants to have advice about how to think and act more con-
structively when the despair comes over her. She has been anxious since she was a child; she has had violent outbursts as long as she can remember. In her mind, it is related to memories that her single mother could not cope with her and occasionally left her, sometimes coming back drunk.

She has had a few short romantic relationships. Usually, they end with Anne getting disappointed over the boyfriend's perceived lack of engagement in her. Anne has been in therapy before. Usually, she has left because she did not feel the therapist gave her the concrete help that she needs.

Anne and her therapist decide that her *problem* is her self-destructive behaviour and her difficulty to rely on others. The *goal* of the treatment will be to help her reduce her self-destructive behaviour and to improve her relational capacity. The focus will be to understand how she can use relationships better for help and support.

In therapy, Anne and her therapist discuss what to do when her urge to cut herself becomes too strong. In addition to attempts to divert the anxiety, they reflect on potential friends to turn to. After some sessions, Anne starts coming late and even not showing up at all. The therapist calls her. When she comes, she says that she feels uncertain whether the therapy method fits her. She wants to have tools for regulating her anxiety. The therapist gives some more suggestions and ideas about how to think and act when she feels an urge to cut herself. In the next session, she tells the therapist that she has cut herself. The tools were of no avail, the anxiety was too strong. The therapist feels disappointed. She suggests that Anne might feel that she is like Anne's mother, unavailable when needed. The next session, Anne has met a young man at a bar, gone home with him, and been raped. The therapist feels pity for her but also feels concern about her carelessness. She considers how to show her reaction. She says that she feels sorry for Anne but cannot help thinking that Anne should have taken care of herself. Anne seems to get hurt and becomes silent. She does not come to the next session.

The therapist again calls her. Anne is hesitant whether to come but de-
cides to do it. At that session, she accuses the therapist for criticizing her for becoming a rape victim. The therapist realizes that she may have been

offensive to Anne and tells her that. Successively, they find ways to discuss their alliance problems.

The therapist's *procedure* in this part of the therapy is to offer concrete suggestions about how to avoid self-destructive behaviour and at the same time explore how Anne can use people for support. When Anne becomes disappointed, the therapist tries to resolve the ruptures that repeatedly occur, and concurrently invite Anne to reflect on the feelings that emerge between them. The *therapeutic process* may be that Anne feels that the therapist genuinely tries to establish a bond with her, and that they successively formulate the feelings that are expressed (and evaded) in the ruptures, thus bringing about reparation of relational damages particularly with regard to trust and reliance on others.

Bertha

Bertha cuts herself when she is angry at herself for not being as successful and attractive as she wants. She, and her mother, has strong expectations that she should be seen as beautiful and intelligent. She becomes particularly stressed when her mother wonders why she has no boyfriend. The mother has great ambitions for her children and drives them as she has driven herself. Bertha does want to be successful and tries to live up to her mother's aspirations. She has a few close friends. Not seldom, she has quarrels with them about petty things that grow to large concerns. She has never had any romantic relationships.

Bertha started therapy at her mother's behest. She talks about her stress of not being able to live up to her mother's ambitions. Her father backs his wife, wishing his daughters to be successful. The therapist gets the impression that Bertha's parents are overly ambitious. When she offers her views about this, Bertha becomes defensive. When listening to Bertha's description of her mother's demands, it seems to the therapist that Bertha needs to become more independent. She tries to be more challenging about whether Bertha has attempted to find her own way. Bertha becomes silent and seems to feel uncertain about what to say. After a few sessions where the therapist tries to encourage Bertha to find her own thoughts about the situation, she realizes that Bertha has become even more avoidant. She discloses that she feels intrusive. Bertha at first avoids also this issue but successively she becomes more critical of the therapist's stance and states that she knows what is best for her.

The *problem* is the self-cutting and, in the therapist's eyes, the tight relationship between mother and daughter. The initial *goal* for the therapy is to help Bertha find other ways to handle the stress. A focus will be to understand the balance between reliance and independence in relation to her mother.

After only a few sessions, the therapist's attempts to question the close relationship between Bertha and her mother seem to fail. Bertha likes her mother and her advice. The more active the therapist becomes, the more silent is Bertha. The therapist suspects that Bertha is more critical than she shows. When asked, she becomes circumstantial but agrees that it is important for her to think about her relationship with her mother. The therapist discloses her frustration at not getting any distinct reaction from Bertha. The next session, Bertha has cut herself. It was rather deep; they had been to the hospital to sew the wound. The therapist realized that the cutting took place on the evening after their last session.

The therapist's *procedure* is to ask Bertha about reactions to her challenges, and to help her become aware of her feelings. The *process* at this stage may be the intensive experience together with the therapist, involving stronger and more varied affects than Bertha is used to, particularly regarding her agency and independence.

Method or perspective?

In the juxtaposition of clinical and theoretical experience from relational psychoanalysis with empirical findings, the question of method or perspective is inevitable. No doubt, most relational therapists consider relational therapy to be a modern version of psychoanalytic therapy. In this sense, relational therapy is a method, possible to compare with other methods.

However, using contemporary research as vantage point, it may be more sensible to consider the relational model as a perspective on psychotherapy. Some head features of a more general relational perspective on psychotherapy are as follows:

- The handling of the process in psychotherapeutic interaction probably has a stronger impact on the results than technical interventions per se. The balance between implicit sensitivity about hardly detectable interactional problems and reflection about them may be crucial.
- Interventions are relational acts. Technical interventions have a contextual relational meaning, they are often relational in nature (admonitions to carry out behavioural and relational experiments, affect attunement, invitations to mentalize about the relationship, roleplaying).
- The therapeutic relationship has personal, emotional meaning for the patient as well as for therapist. The personal significance is mutual; if the relationship matters to the patient, it matters to the therapist also. It is, for instance, hard to conceive of corrective emotional experiences as being effective if the patient has not become emotionally important to the therapist.
- The mutual therapeutic work moves in the dialectics between exploring and understanding the patient's history and aligning with his forward-oriented directionality.

With this view of therapy, focus on the relationship is a perspective on therapy. In any treatment form, the focus can be redirected from techniques to the actual therapeutic relationship. Not that techniques of various kinds should not be useful, but they are implemented in a relational context, and aspects of this context often have a curative significance. In every engaged relationship, the partners by and by realize that what happens between them has importance for the solution of the task they set out with. The therapist's mind set can be seen as the agent of change (Seligman, 2014).

7 Affects, attachment, and mentalizing in the therapeutic relationship

Several aspects of the therapeutic relationship have particular importance for treatment outcome. Among them are affects, attachment, and mentalizing. These are often seen as individual capacities, possible to categorize or rate as personality traits. However, they develop in relationships, come to life in relationships, and can readily be seen as defining aspects of relationships. They are significant examples of the intricate interplay between the individuals' life experiences and the emergent nature of the interaction.

Affects

Affects are the driving energy in human relationships. Although neuroimaging has greatly expanded the knowledge of the neural substrates for affects, the hope that such studies would enrich our understanding of the meaning and experience of feelings has basically come to naught (Gazzaniga, 2015). Are affects biologically and evolutionary distinct or are they socially construed? The issue has importance as relational constructionism presupposes co-created understanding of the ongoing emotional interplay.

The *basic emotions theories* contend that there is a limited number of easily recognized distinct affects that have evolutionary meaning and specific biological substrates (Ekman, 1992; Tomkins, 1962–1963, 1991). The specific neurophysiological substratum defines the emotion. If the neurological circuit producing a certain affect is active, the emotion is active, whether the individual feels it or not. The differences between emotions are functional as they serve specific purposes. The propensity to experience them is innate; they have evolved as useful tools for survival. Expressions of them are similar in different cultures and also among newborns and primates.

The *appraisal theory* states that although emotions have distinct neurological patterns, the experience of them is coloured by culture and individual experiences. Emotions are not categorical but exist on continua. Perception of emotions depend on social context, personality, and current goals (Ellsworth, 2013; Frijda, 1986).

A third theory of emotions consider them to be *psychological constructions*, created by the person in response to the current context (Barrett, 2017). Each

DOI: 10.4324/9781003026914-7

experience of sadness has a new shape, a specific granularity. Subjective reports are the only way to understand an emotion.

Finally, *social constructionism* considers emotions to be created in the social context. A person's emotion concepts are based on the goals of the culture (Mesquita, Boiger, & De Leersnyder, 2016). In what way a person constructs an emotional experience depends on its social consequences, they can be seen as "emotional discourses" (Averill, 2012).

In the basic emotions theory (Ekman, Campos, Davidson, & de Wall, 2003; Tomkins, 1991), primary emotions are thought to come quickly, have short duration, and to be appraised immediately. Jurist (2018), on the contrary, argues that feelings may be hard to discover and to distinguish. Some persons have permanent difficulties to access and name feelings (alexithymia); most people have situational and occasional problems of naming their ongoing feeling state.

The relational perspective on emotions is to underline their significance for the evolvement of relationships and the mutuality in accessing and interpreting them. For practical reasons, a "dyadic emotional discourse" model fits this perspective.

Affects in therapy

Affects are central to change in most therapy methods (Greenberg, 2008). Some methods emphasize the need to learn how to regulate affects, other methods focus on the need for the patient to tolerate and not avoid affects. In affect-focused dynamic therapies, the idea is that the patient needs to explore layers of inhibiting, secondary feelings in order to contact more primary and liberating feelings. These therapies focus on the patient's awareness, modulation, and expression of affects.

In addition to this goal, the relational therapist also uses her own feelings, actively, openly, and mindfully. A basic task in therapy is to transform sensational innuendos to affects. "Every time a patient and analyst can each access and openly share their dissociated affective experience of something that is taking place between them—some cognitively unsymbolizable aspect of their mutual experience that is felt but is unthinkable—the process of state-sharing through which this takes place begins to enlarge the domain and fluency of the dialogue" (Bromberg, 2011, p. 136).

The issue of how to become aware of affects, and what kind of affective awareness the patient and the therapist are open for, is central. Not all affects are discrete. Stern (1985) described vitality affects as background emotional states, Damasio (1999, 2010) called similar affective states "primordial feelings", and Ferro (2011) used the concept "proto-emotions". Jurist (2018) uses the term aporetic emotions, meaning an emotional state where discrete emotions are hard to distinguish. Although with different theoretical emphases, these ideas suggest that feelings may be vaguely felt and unclear to their nature. This may be the most common emotional position; the mind monitors the body for indicators of a feeling state, basically in terms of valence (pleasure and pain) and degree of arousal, until a clear and distinct feeling emerges.

The therapist's emotional avoidance

Affect-focused therapies focus on encouraging patients to remain in affect states and not to avoid them. The idea is similar to anxiety exposure; when the affect is experienced fully, it will be transformed to something else: another feeling, another body sensation. In relational therapy, the same stance is necessary for the therapist: to stay in the feeling, to tolerate it, to wait for its transformation. It will not disappear, but it will change.

Sometimes, management of countertransference feelings is supposed to imply that the therapist regulates her feelings, puts them in context in order to make them less intense (Hayes, Gelso, Goldberg, & Kivlighan, 2018). This is a defensive stance. Using the therapist's affects requires that they are genuine, and with adequate intensity. If the therapist feels strong warmth and sympathy for her patient, let it remain as long as it does; if the therapist hates her patient, continue hating until the hate becomes transformed. Avoided affects tend to stay; tolerated feelings change. The therapeutic skill is to be aware of the changes, not to cling to the feeling when it moves, not to be programmatic or normative about the therapist's emotional stance.

Attachment

Attachment is the mammal toddler's way of securing life and food by keeping close to the caregiver (Bowlby, 1969). Depending on the character of the infant-caregiver relationship, different patterns of attachment evolve. Developmental research shows that these interactional patterns become internalized in the infant as "inner working models". In new relationships, these patterns are used to regulate the person's feelings of vulnerability and security in relation to the other.

Bowlby's understanding of maternal deprivation of the child's needs as a main cause of mental problems was dismissed by psychoanalysts of his time (Bowlby, 1969; Fonagy & Campbell, 2015). The relational movement has embraced attachment theory (Mitchell, 2000; Mitchell & Aron, 1999; Wallin, 2007) but has been sceptical about the usefulness of systematic studies of attachment (Hoffman, 2009b).

Attachment security is closely related to the caregiver's mentalizing about their offspring. Fonagy, Steele, and Steel (1991) found that children of mothers with better mentalizing ability during pregnancy had more securely attached toddlers. Thus, parental mental states influence infant attachment organization (Main, Goldwyn & Hesse, 2003).

Attachment patterns and therapist reactions

Studies suggest that the creation of attachment is dyadic, between parent and child and also between therapist and patient (Beebe et al., 2010, p. 113; Fonagy & Campbell, 2015). Usually, however, there is an imbalance. "The therapist inevitably is pulled to provide the complementary response because the client is more adept, more expert in his distinctive, rigid, and extreme game of interpersonal encounter... The therapist cannot *not* be hooked temporarily into providing the complementary response to the client" (Kiesler, 1986, p. 14).

Patients with dismissive attachment may make the therapist feel super-fluous, insufficient, and perhaps intrusive and evoke feelings of emptiness. Sometimes, these patients evoke idealized feelings as a way to keep distance to genuine relating (Daniel, 2015; Wallin, 2007; Westerling et al., 2019). Patients with an anxious/ambivalent attachment may initially evoke sympathy and warmth, but successively the therapist may feel overwhelmed and unfree, perhaps insufficient. Some of these patients may evoke a therapist tendency to take care and sometimes also erotic feelings. The disorganized patient often evokes confused and sometimes scaring feelings (Holmes & Slade, 2018).

Is the therapeutic relationship an attachment relationship?

It has been argued that the therapy relationship is an attachment relation-ship. The therapist offers a secure base and a safe haven. The patient may feel safe while exploring new relational possibilities. Attachment deficiencies can be repaired through experiences in relationship (Pearlman & Courtois, 2005). Mikulincer, Shaver, and Berant (2013) gave five reasons for con-sidering the therapy relationship as an attachment relationship: (1) the therapist is perceived as more skilled, (2) the patient seeks help, (3) the therapy is perceived as a secure base and (4) haven, and (5) the patient fears the separation. Using the Patient Attachment Coding System (PACS), Talia, Miller-Bottome, and Daniel (2017) found that secure attachment in relation to the therapist was associated with more repaired alliance ruptures (Miller-Bottome, Talia, Safran, & Muran, 2018).

Therapists should be aware both of the great potential of improving at-tachment security in therapy and of the risk of idealizing the relationship in attachment terms as being more significant than it actually is.

Mentalizing

Mentalizing can be described as the ability to know the difference between an organism with intentions and a stone, to know that humans have a complicated and opaque mental life that is not directly understandable from the individual's behaviour. Thoughts, feelings, and fantasies are not directly shown in behaviour, there are even aspects of a person's own mental life that he is not aware of. Mentalizing is the ability to tolerate uncertainty about underlying motives and intentions. This is self-evident once we know it, we do not even think of it. It is, however, a developmental achievement, attained by most children around four.

Mentalizing, like attachment, is understood as an individual ability. However, mentalizing is shared. Although an individual may reflect on different motives and meanings of his own or others' behaviour, mentalizing develops and is maintained by other's reflections, comments, and actions.

Both explicit and implicit mentalizing can be classified or scored as a social competence. Intensive emotional states or permanent personality dysfuntion may reduce a person's mentalizing capacity (Fonagy, Gergely, Jurist, & Target, 2002). In ordinary life, and in therapy, we move between degrees of mentalizing. It would be unbearable to constantly reflect on various aspects of our own and others' minds.

Dimensions of mentalizing

Mentalizing may be the explicit, conscious ability to reflect about oneself, others, and relationships in an attentive, nuanced, open-minded way, and it may also be the implicit, automatic, immediate, unreflective, procedural, and often non-verbal ability to know how to relate to others, a process that "requires little or no attention, intention or awareness and effort" (Bateman & Fonagy 2012, p. 20). These stances may gradually move into each other. In a new relationship, a person may actively reflect on the other's intentions and feelings, and on her own. This attention successively wanes, the person gets habituated to the other's reactions and to her own reactions to her. However, a sudden change in the other's attitude can awaken new curiosity on the other and on oneself.

Psychic equivalence

The child is afraid of the scorpion in his bed. The mother tries to reassure the boy by searching the bed, shaking the blanket, shining with a torch. "Do you feel certain now that there is no scorpion?" "Yes, but when you turn off the light, it will be back". What is in the mind becomes physical reality.

Psychic equivalence means that the distinction between imagination and reality has collapsed. The inner world is not separated from the outer, concrete world. Thoughts are concrete truths. The prototypical example is the depressed person's conviction that her depressive thoughts cannot be questioned.

There are many ways to end up in psychological equivalence in psychological treatment. Not uncommon is to understand the patient's problems as caused by a diagnosis or a particular event. We are certain that ADHD or the fact that his father used to beat him accounts for the patient's inattention. We apply the physical cause-effect schema and leave the reflecting stance.

Pretend mode

If the psychic equivalence mode implies an exaggerated reliance on the truth that the mental world creates, its opposite is the pretend mode. In the pretend mode, the mental life has no real connection with the external reality. Being in love without any move to let the love change the practical life can be pretend mode, as can talking about getting a divorce without ever taking any steps in that direction.

Sometimes, psychotherapy becomes pretend mode. The patient and the therapist can pretend therapy, sometimes seemingly indefinitely. There may be a temptation for the therapist as well as for the patient to feel that the subject being reflected on is highly important and meaningful although no real therapeutic work is made.

The teleological stance

Sometimes, words must be followed by action. But there are occasions when the mental world does not have to translate to action. To trust a person does not have to be confirmed by a paper or a hug. In the teleological mode, however, action is what counts. "So, he had strong suicide thoughts? Did he make any attempt? If not, probably it was just a show". In the teleological stance, the person cannot understand the intention or feelings of another person if they are not expressed as actions. The person needs sexual intercourse to be certain that his partner loves him.

Mentalizing in the therapeutic relationship

To help patients improve their mentalizing capacity is a significant goal in many therapies, also in relational therapy. Mentalizing is an important ability for using psychotherapy. Mentalizing patients make better use of interpretative interventions in comparison with support in short-term psychodynamic therapy (Cromer & Hilsenroth, 2010; Piper, Joyce, McCallum, & Azim, 1998). These patients also create stronger alliance and improve more in short-term therapy (Bressi et al., 2017; Ekeblad, Falkenström, & Holmqvist, 2016).

It is natural to use the therapeutic relationship for improving mentalizing. An important therapist skill is to adjust the relationship in order to increase its potential for mentalizing.

Patients with disorganized attachment may lose their mentalizing capacity if they feel threatened about their attachment security (Bateman & Fonagy, 2016).

Talking therapies imply a special risk that the therapy becomes a pretend mode project. Patient and therapist may meet to deepen their understanding of the patient's problems, talk about their relationship, although nothing happens in the patient's relationships outside therapy. To assess the usefulness of the therapy is a delicate task. The patient's mental world may change without much visible indications. On the other hand, therapies that focus on behaviour change do not seem to increase patients' mentalizing ability, whereas therapies that assist patients in developing better understanding of interpersonal problems do (Ekeblad, Falkenström, & Holmqvist, 2016; Rudden, Milrod, Target, Ackerman, & Graf, 2006).

8 Support and challenge

In this practice section, distinct features of a relational approach to therapy and illustrations of how to use them are presented. Before the presentation of the case and the tools, some general reflections on therapeutic practice will be made. In this chapter, the balance between support and challenge is discussed.

Most therapies have supportive and challenging elements. Supportive may imply that the therapist encourages constructive activities and ways of thinking that the patient already has developed and uses. It can also mean that the therapist confirms and validates the patient's reactions and ways of thinking as understandable. Such interventions are often thought of as verbal support for the patient's reactions. A more relational understanding is to use the therapeutic interaction for validating the patient's capacities. Consider the emotionally inhibited patient who finds it hard to be open with his partner. In the therapy, he has become confidential with her therapist. He tries to find the words for it. The therapist also strives to find the right expressions for the closeness that has evolved. By meta-communicating about her own problems to find the right words, and perhaps timidity about formulating them, she validates the patient's experience.

The therapist challenges the patient when she questions his way of thinking, feeling, or behaving; encourages him to think, feel, or behave in new ways; try new approaches, or perhaps dare him to do things that may arouse unpleasant feelings.

In relational therapy, challenge is shared. The therapist challenges the patient by inviting him to be as open as possible about painful memories and experiences. He or he may also challenge him to tolerate anxiety and to alter behaviour. Some patients "can be helped to alter behavior, and [only then be brought] to introspective insight ... changing patterns of behavior and activity can provide opportunities for insight" (Trop, Burke, & Trop, 2002; pp. 219–220). This is of course true. In relational therapy, the point is not, however, the effects of behavioural experiments per se but the negotiations around them. The darkness-fearing child in Chapter 1 illustrates how attempts to persuade the patient may provide material.

The therapist also challenges himself or herself. By earnestly commenting on the ongoing interaction, he or she makes herself vulnerable for the patient's

DOI: 10.4324/9781003026914-8

reactions. Instead of avoiding comments about the interaction by arguing that the patient is too fragile, vulnerable, or impulsive, he or she exposes herself to unknown reactions. The relational challenge for the therapist is to tolerate uncertainty, to walk on thin ice, to explore hassles and conflicts in the therapeutic relationship, and to make himself or herself vulnerable.

An illustration:

The patient has been offered a severance payment if he quits his job as a salesman. There are conflicts at his job, but the therapist does not have a clear picture of them. The patient does not want to leave his work; he is afraid that he will remain unemployed. The therapist has thought about what it might be like to work with the patient. She hears him talking about conflicts with colleagues, but it is unclear who initiates them and how they are sorted out. She can imagine that there are workmates who get irritated on him, but she feels uncertain whether they harass him. Her own experience is that the patient can sometimes be overly categorical about things. In those instances, she feels quite frustrated with him.

A supportive intervention:

- I know you get angry from time to time at your fellow workers.
- Well, yes it happens. They think rules can be broken at will. I do get annoyed.
- I guess you're not the only one who does. But I have heard you react in different ways. Although you sometimes seem to get quite mad at them, at other times, you are rather in a negotiating mood. You think that's more helpful for you?
- Sometimes I do get angry. But then I try to calm down as soon as possible.
- In our work, I have appreciated when we get curious together and use it for learning about ourselves.

A challenging intervention:

- I know you get angry from time to time at your fellow workers. You're in a problematic situation. Your boss wants to fire you. Is that because of conflicts with your colleagues?
- He says I'm a troublemaker. Just because I want to be fair to all.
- I can't know, of course. But I've thought about us. Last time I had the feeling that you wanted me to agree with you in your complaints. Afterwards I realized that I felt kind of forced, like I lost my space to reflect.
- Don't you think I'm right? Do you think I should take anything?
- No. But something happens here. You want me to agree about something that I don't know anything about.
- Of course not, but I've told you how it is there.

- That's true but right now I'd like to explore what's happening here between us. I felt a sting of irritation about your attitude.
- You want to drive home that I'm an awkward type.
- The therapist continues by describing that at times she feels frustrated in her attempts to see situations from different perspectives. The patient becomes angry and disappointed, the therapist has a touch of bad conscience but continues to describe her impressions. The patient becomes more silent, the therapist experiences him as sulky.
- Did I get us into an impasse? I felt it was important for me to describe my impression of you. Guess I was afraid you wouldn't take it in.
- No problem, I've heard it before.

In an oft-cited statement, Freud recommended the therapist to model the technique on "the surgeon, who puts aside all his feelings, even his human sympathy" (Freud, 1912a, p. 115). Although written in a specific context, it illustrates Freud's basic ambition: exploration of repressed mental content. In contrast, Ferenczi in his papers from the 1930s advocated an approach where the therapist shows appreciation, sympathy, and even love to his patient. The conflict between explorative and affirmative approaches is alive to this day, here called challenge and support.

Empathy

The ability to see the world from the patient's perspective, to resonate with his feelings, and to express this understanding in a helpful way is an important therapist competence. It has the potential to be both supportive and challenging.

Two psychotherapy pioneers, Rogers and Kohut, both highlighted the importance of empathy (Bohart, 1991; Kahn & Rachman, 2000). Rogers' idea was that what the patient says is right but needs elaboration. The goal is to help him formulate his feelings and hopes more clearly. Kohut also successively turned to the idea that what the patient says is right, "profound", whereas the therapist's own interpretations may be "superficial" (Kohut, 1984). Kohut's perspective was developmental and reparative; empathy is a means to cure the patient's self-image damages. Kohut saw empathy as the basic therapeutic intervention, a transformative mechanism for healing the patient's narcissistic wounds (Kohut, 1959), with more and more of a caring intention (Kahn, 1985).

For Rogers, empathy is a way of actualizing the patient's dormant potential. Rogers had a "romantic" view of man as an individual with potential, forward-directed, whereas Kohut emphasized a more "tragic" view of man's situation as repeatedly abandoned.

In the perspective of relational therapy, both Rogers and Kohut are one-person theorists. The focus is squarely on the patient. The therapist's task is to liberate the patient's self, to help remove inhibitions and restrictions. From a relational standpoint, two aspects are particularly important; the subjectivity of the empathizer and the issue of with whom the therapist empathizes.

The empathizer

To know something about someone else is conditioned on knowing something about oneself. The idea that understanding the other's feelings, thoughts, and motives presupposes some understanding of oneself has, interestingly, support in Webster's definition of empathy: "projection of one's own personality onto the personality of another of one's own emotions, responses etc. in order to understand them better" (1966, p. 457).

However, all therapists have not been depressed or had anxiety attacks, all therapists do not have disorganized attachment, all therapists have not had traumatic childhoods. How is it possible to understand someone else who struggles with problems that the therapist has not experienced? One answer is that empathy is not a state, it is a process (Pao, 1983). In the process from the immediate reaction to the other's predicament to a more complex understanding of the other's situation, the empathizer uses her mental resources to come closer to the patient's experience (Stern, 1994).

Even a narrative about torture or abuse comes in a relational context; a prior conversational exchange leads up to the patient's telling the story and the way it is told. No story is told out of context, all conversation has a relational meaning and influences the mutual understanding. In this process, the empathizer uses her experience and imagination, she places what she hears in her own mental landscape.

"You don't understand me!" The patient may want the therapist not only to sympathize with his experience, but to see the world through his eyes. The therapist offers suggestions about how to understand his father's egocentric style, but the understanding is felt as insufficient. The therapist feels caught in her lack of accurate understanding, unable to move in her own mental universe. She tries ever new ideas. The patient feels half by half understood, they move in some way towards a common image, but the split is still there. In this process, the patient recognizes the therapist's and his own subjectivity. Empathy is a movement, with halts and steps forward.

The Boston BCPSG offers this description of the therapist's position: "The process of moving through and being moved by another involves the implicit 'trying on' of the other's subtle differences in attitude toward the self and toward other important relationships in one's life. The implicit 'trying on' of another's orientation, in turn, creates an implicit pull to integrate that other's 'take' on the world with one's own, with resulting struggle and potential reorganization of previous experience" (BCPSG, 2018b, p. 300). Empathy is a negotiation process, with attempts to understand, debacles, and new attempts.

Not only does the empathizer try on the experiences of the other; she also let them change her. Buber (1923) emphasized that in the mutual I–Thou relationship, both participants are changed. In seeing the uniqueness of the other, the meeting becomes transformative for both.

The attention that empathy implies may at times have a profound influence on the other (Aragno, 2008). There is a dialectical relationship between empathy and recognition. In empathy, one person tries to identify with, take the position of the other. Recognition, in contrast, means that the two individuals are felt as separate, retaining their separateness. As a part of the child's development, it may need to be completely understood by the parent, but it may also need to recognize the separateness of the other, and to be known in its own separateness (McKay, 2019). Interestingly, this perspective on serious human relating, the other's separateness, was developed by the other great 20th-century Jewish philosopher, Levinas (1972).

With whom does the therapist empathize?

The psychoanalytic concept "technical neutrality" carries the hope that the therapist may be open to and identify with different aspects of the patient's internal world. The kind person who feels deceived may harbor aggressive fantasies that remain in the shadows if the therapist is too eager to identify with the deceived aspect. The therapist's ambition is to be available for all aspects of the patient's self.

A less reticent and more interactionally active therapist may end up in identifications with the most visible aspects of the patient. One part of the patient's self-system may attract one aspect of the therapist's self, leading to collusion and loss of availability for other parts. As noted previously, this is the condition and the risk, in engaged interaction. One of the dilemmas in relational therapy is to move between excessive empathy with limited aspects of the patient and attempts to reach an observational, reflective position.

9 Recipes and tools

Therapy methods these days often come with treatment manuals and guidelines, sometimes step-by-step recommendations. The quest for verified outcome results requires that the treatment method is defined, and definition often means a manual. Relational therapy is characterized by openness, uncertainty, spontaneity, and "sloppiness" (Hoffman, 2006). However, even if such thoughts may be enticing, therapists need more concrete ideas of how to do (Davies, 2018). Throwing away the book does not mean that anything goes. Some approaches are more relational than other.

Tools

To describe therapy methods as tools or strategies is common in solution-focused treatments. Tools are used to improve or change something. A rake, a grater, a planer. In a treatment context, a tool may be mindfulness meditation, or a thought that the patient can use in stressful or challenging situations. "Don't take over someone else's job!" may be a good recommendation to an overburdened person. The therapist offers the tool, and the patient uses it.

In the relational perspective, tools are primarily used by the therapist. It is not even certain that the patient is aware that a tool is used. When the therapist endeavours to "stay in the present, to be concrete and specific", the patient probably does not observe it as a tool.

Relational interventions are attempts. They are made with the best will and understanding, but with the uncertainty that characterizes engagement in personal conversations. The core of relational therapy is to be attentive to the interaction (Seligman, 2014), to note gaps and hassles, to allow certainty to become ambiguous or unclear and the emotions to surprise us, and to be open to genuine, transformative talk.

The patient's experience and the therapist's expertise

In 1961, Jerome Frank suggested that all treatments for mental problems have a common underlying structure. According to Frank, successful therapy always goes through a four-stage process. The first step is to

DOI: 10.4324/9781003026914-9

establish a trustful contact with the patient, the second to give the patient hope that change is possible, on the third, the therapist gives the patient a credible explanation of the problem, and on the fourth, the therapist uses her therapeutic procedure (Frank & Frank, 1993).

The core of this idea is that the therapist must understand the patient's mental, social, and cultural context. Therapists heal patients by using methods that are credible to them. The therapist's expertise must fit into the patient's cultural and personal experience. The model points to the balance between the two. Most therapy schools emphasize the therapist's expertise. In contrast, Bohart (2000) suggests that "clients are the active self-healing agents in therapy, aided and abetted by the therapist, who supplies the chair. Techniques are tools or prostheses clients use in their self-healing efforts, and therapy is ultimately the provision of support and structure for naturally occurring client self-healing processes" (p. 130).

The question of the balance between the therapist's expertise and the patient's experience is crucial in understanding psychological change. Relational theory emphasizes not only the combination, but often the clash, between the patient's and the therapist's perspectives.

The balance between therapist expertise and patient experience is subtle to uphold theoretically. An example is the rupture-resolution model (Safran & Muran, 2000) which, although open for analyzing the interaction and for granting the therapist's contribution to ruptures, basically assumes that the therapist uses defined procedures for resolving problems, and for reaching specific goals.

Another take on this issue is presented by the communication systems therapy model (Allison & Fonagy, 2016; Fonagy & Allison, 2014; Fonagy, Luyten, & Allison, 2015). Fonagy and colleagues argue that successful psychological treatment depends on the therapist's ability to make her model of treatment believable in the patient's eyes. According to these authors, a basic characteristic of early human interaction is the need for the child to have somebody to trust for acquiring social knowledge. As the time for cognitive and emotional maturation is longer among humans than among other primates, the human child needs to trust its caregivers. If the child has a secure attachment to the parent, it develops "epistemic trust" in her. In order for therapy to work, the patient needs to have epistemic trust in the therapist. Therapies, in this model, passes three steps or "systems".

The therapist sees the patient

On the first step, the therapist shows curiosity about the patient, his situation, and his attempts to handle his problems. This is an explorative, negotiating stage. The therapist's task is to listen with interest and engagement to the patient's solution attempts and, at the same time, offer her own thoughts about how the problems can be handled. If the patient understands that the therapist is curious about him and his ways of handling the problems, it becomes possible for her to suggest measures that seem reasonable in the patient's eyes. For the model to work, the patient must understand that the therapist perceives him as a person who can do something about his or her situation. It is likely easier for the patient to trust the therapist if she has a clear model for how change can be achieved (Benish, Imel & Wampold, 2008; Fonagy & Allison, 2014; Leichsenring et al., 2015; McAleavey & Castonguay, 2014).

The restoration of robust mentalization

At the second step in this model, the therapist's confidence in the patient's ability to deal with his or her problems enables the patient to start thinking more openly about opportunities to address the problems. The patient's mentalizing capacity increases. He starts seeing himself as a person who can do something about his difficulties, with skills to cope with them. Fonagy and Allison (2014) underscore that the primary purpose is not to improve the patient's mentalizing capacity per se, but to help him use his mentalizing ability to become curious about his social and relational surroundings. This may happen if the patient develops epistemic trust in the therapist, if he finds himself in the therapist's mind.

The therapist and the patient negotiations can be described like this from the therapist's perspective:

– I hope that you see me as a credible person, and that my suggestions to become curious in other relationships are meaningful and helpful for you.

And from the patient's:

– When you see me as a person who can change my social behaviour, I can see myself in the same way.

The revival of social learning

To be understood is a prerequisite for the patient to be able to begin mentalizing. As he begins to be curious about himself and others, he understands himself better. He starts noticing interest from others and feels understood by others. As the patient begins to feel that others are interested in him and cares for him, interest in social contacts increases. A positive relational circle has been started. This leads to a decrease in epistemic vigilance. The patient begins to trust others and what they say. This leads to "recovery of the capacity for social information exchange that … is at the heart of effective psychotherapies" (Fonagy & Allison, 2014, p. 377).

The communication model, like the rupture-resolution model, gives full respect to the patient's experiences. However, with a relational perspective, it retains the idea that there are specific procedures that the therapist should use to reach a goal. Relational therapy has an even more open view of the therapist's procedural approaches.

Structure of the practice chapters

In this section on relational practice, the same structure will be used in each chapter. A short description of the intervention, called tool, will be followed by a presentation of the purpose of the tool and a potential dilemma in using the tool. After a description of the theoretical principles comes a vignette from a therapy that will be followed in all chapters. A section on practical recommendations ends each chapter.

There is in the therapy literature a tendency to present dramatic cases and amazing moments in the sessions. "Despite their feel for the analyst–patient interaction, relational reports sometimes highlight a crucial moment of impasse and its resolution, perhaps at the expense of all the everyday, in- cremental routine that precedes and follows those moments" (Seligman, 2014, p. 649). The cases and dialogues presented in this practice section are close to everyday routine clinical practice.

Part II

Practices

10 David

David is a man of 45 with recurring depressions and panic attacks. For long periods, he loses all energy and has suicidal thoughts. He has been on sick leave for several rounds and at present he has been home for four months. His psychiatric diagnoses are melancholic depression and personality syndrome not otherwise specified.

He has received treatments of different kinds and with varying success. He has tried several medications, such as lithium and antidepressants. He has been recommended ECT but refused. In the most ambitious psychological treatment so far, his therapist used a CBT approach, mainly trying to motivate him to become more physically and socially active. They also made some cognitive work, focusing on monitoring situations when his depressive and suicidal thoughts peaked and to write down his thoughts and feelings at those moments. Although he really tried, he did not get any better, and after a while he became less motivated to perform the tasks. He thinks that part of the cause for his problems is genetic. Several persons in his family have had nervous problems.

Sometimes David drinks too much. He has used Antabuse previously, but he does not want to get any help for alcohol abuse; in his view, he does not drink more than he can stand.

David has been married for 12 years with Carin. They have three children, now nine, seven and four. David says he loves Carin, and he is anxious about their relationship. But when he feels down and apathetic, he does not stand listening to her or to be with her. He wishes that he could, but he prefers to be on his own, lying on the couch looking at TV. Although he is usually a kind person, he may flare up towards his wife and his children, sometimes even becoming rough towards the children. There is a notification of concern about him at the social service office, submitted by parents of his children's peers.

He has worked for several years at an auto garage. It is quite a small place, and the employees know each other well. David likes his boss, but he does not always tolerate his work mates. In particular, he has problems with

DOI: 10.4324/9781003026914-10

Inga, a young colleague. He thinks she tries to denigrate him with her newer knowledge from school. He does not know if Inga knows about his irritation at her and he does not want to come in conflict with her. He admits that she knows quite a lot about diagnosing car problems with the computer and he recognizes that he is envious of her.

The garage was previously owned by his uncle. David's father left the family when he was three and shortly afterwards committed suicide. His uncle became a kind of backup father to him. His mother worked in the cash register at a movie theatre, usually in the evenings. Those days, he was with the uncle and the uncle's wife, David's aunt. They have three children. David is the same age as their middle child, Lisa. As an adult, he has often thought about how they treated him. He was in no way maltreated; on the contrary, they were always careful that he should participate as much as their own children. But everyone knew that when they talked about more long-term things, such as holidays or where to celebrate Christmas, he was not included.

His mother certainly liked him a lot and she did her best to make life ok for him, at home and with his uncle. Sometimes she met other men. David felt they were important to her, and he did not want to complicate things for her when she wanted to be with them. These relationships were often short, and he seldom got to know the men. One man stayed for quite some time and a couple of times they went on vacation all three. Peter was nice to David and David became attached to him. Sometimes, he thought he would tell Peter that he wanted mom and him to marry but he never dared. Towards the end of the relationship, Peter and his mother quarreled a lot and David understood that it might come to an end.

When his mother was lonely, she sometimes drank too much. A few times, David went to his uncle and told him that his mother was drunk. Once, his uncle took her to a hospital. She remained there for a week and during this time, David stayed with his uncle. When she got home, everything was as usual. He never talked with his mother about these events.

His wife is positive about his treatment. But she is tired of David never getting better and she has the impression that he does not use the therapy in the best way. She appreciated when he was encouraged to become more active, and she thinks he gave up too easily. She looks forward to the visit from the social secretary; she wants to have a serious talk about what happens between David and the children. She hopes he will get help for his drinking.

His therapist Anne is about ten years younger than David. She lives with her husband. They have no children but have recently decided to try to get one. Anne defines her method as relational. She has been trained in several other treatment methods and is happy to combine techniques from different schools. She tries to use the ongoing relationship with the patient in a more active way than she did previously. She gets supervision in relational therapy.

11 Try to understand who the patient is

The tool

How do you get to know a person, his perspective on the world, his life struggles, his specific form of suffering? To know in depth takes time but the first impression is valuable. Since we easily get stuck in old tracks with each other, the first meetings are golden opportunities to discover the unusual and unexpected. Once we get used to each other, it becomes more difficult to see what stands out.

The image I create of a person will differ from others' images. This is particularly true if my images grow in a contact where others' impressions do not modify them. The therapy situation is intended to give the patient opportunity to present himself on his own terms. But it also means that the image is limited by the dyadic frames that the therapy situation usually entails.

It may be important to know if a patient has a psychiatric diagnosis, a specific attachment pattern, particular types of relational difficulties. But this rarely says very much about who the person is. It is striking how advance information about a person often is felt as irrelevant once you meet him. In the real meeting, the person comes forth with unique traits, habits, ways of talking, interest in understanding what happens in the interaction, and capacity to tolerate suffering.

Sometimes it may be useful to ask patients to describe themselves with self-assessment forms and in formalized interviews. However, the therapist should realize that answers to questionnaires and interviews come in a context. The patient knows that they will have significance for the therapist's image of him. The patient's responses are not objective reports of thoughts and feelings but communications about them to the therapist and attempts to give the therapist a picture of him. The patient creates relation with his words.

Relational treatment is not about creating a good relationship with the patient, but to encourage curiosity about how the relationship is experienced and can be used. The aim is not to be perceived as kind and friendly, but to show interest in how the patient understands his world, ant to pay attention to what happens in the interaction.

DOI: 10.4324/9781003026914-11

The purpose

The purpose of getting to know the patient is to get a sense for how his need for help can be understood in his life context and whether the therapist can help him. It is important to be open to the complexity of the patient's image of himself and realize that many aspects of him cannot be formulated. The general principle in all treatment: to first diagnose or systematically describe the patient's problems and then begin the treatment is in a trivial sense also valid for relational treatment. But in reality, the understanding of the patient's troubles will be nuanced and reformulated successively during the therapy; that is one of the aims of the therapy.

It is important to understand in what way the context where treatment takes place creates expectations. Some patients have an instrumental view; they want to hear what diagnosis they have and if the therapist has the skills to deal with such conditions. The therapist's response may have to combined with descriptions about how relational treatment works, and in some way describe the difference between a medical and a contextual perspective on therapy. The patient should have the chance to choose a more symptom-focused treatment.

The therapist should also get a feeling for what it is like to work with the patient, what interventions might be useful and what issues may be hard to deal with. The assessment is a test treatment. Starting a relational treatment is not just about choice of method, it is equally about choice of person and choice of ways of being together. The empirical evidence for a constructive therapy is tied to the fit between patient and therapist (Wampold & Imel, 2015).

The dilemma

Every person carries his life history, his relationship patterns and skills, and his personality weaknesses and strengths, perhaps even a psychiatric diagnosis. When meeting another person, some of these characteristics emerge, others remain in the background. During a longer contact with a person, the understanding of the person's individuality may come into a new light. The interaction gives colour to certain aspects of the person. In emotionally charged contacts, dimensions of the patient may emerge that are not always obvious at the start.

The dyadic interaction is an important aspect of relational assessment. The contrast between the "general" patient and the patient in the therapeutic relationship with a specific therapist creates a dilemma when it comes to making an assessment. Assessments in the healthcare system should not depend on who makes them. With reason we get upset when different physicians make different assessments of the same somatic condition.

A relational view of assessment means that throughout the process it is based on the relationship we create with the patient. Admittedly, scores and ratings on formalized interview assessments can enrich the picture. But assessments take place in a social and cultural context and are influenced by the interaction in the assessment relationship. The dilemma of relational treatment assessments is the tension between the potential interest in a factual and "impartial" assessment and the fact that our assessments of other people and their concerns are always subjectively, or rather inter-subjectively, intertwined.

Principles

Diagnoses and evaluations

Questions about diagnosis and psychological dysfunction often come soon in a therapist's head these days. Does the patient have autistic traits? Should his way of using his cell phone be considered dependence in a diagnostic sense? Perhaps he has an avoidant attachment style? Therapists and patients live in a social world where diagnoses are bread and butter in newspapers and social conversations.

In somatic medicine, distinctions are made between diagnoses based on objective findings and anamnestic diagnoses. A cancer tumour is assessed on the type of mutations the cells have made; pneumonia can be established on pathogenic bacteria. In some conditions, no objective findings are made; the diagnoses are anamnestic. People may have back pain without any physiological cause. In such cases, the diagnosis is based on the patient's medical history and subjective report. But attempts are always made to find physical causes; the scientific model assumes that there is one. There is always a causal presumption.

Psychiatric diagnoses are never based on objective lab findings. They are based on the patient's own story, descriptions by family and friends or observations of the patient's behaviour. They are not presumed to be causal; they are categories of symptoms. Sometimes, diagnoses change over time without obvious scientific progress. The arguments around the hysteria diagnosis, described by Hippocrates and used by Charcot and Freud, speak for its arbitrariness as do diagnoses of sexual behaviour.

Relational treatment has evolved from theories and clinical contexts that are not interested in psychiatric and psychological diagnoses and assessments. Many authors look at them with distrust (Hoffman, 2009a). There are no relational intervention programmes for symptoms or syndromes. The emphasis on the patient's unique life history and on the importance of the jointly created understanding means that diagnoses and other judgements based on categorizing people by behaviours and disorders do not fit well in the model. This scepticism about the utility of psychiatric assessment is not unique to relational therapy. In many other forms of treatment, there is also a scepticism about symptom- and diagnosis-based assessments (Barlow & Kennedy, 2016; Hofmann & Hayes, 2019).

It is suggestive to read what Carl Rogers, one of the first empirical psychotherapy researchers, wrote about diagnoses:

> When one thinks of the vast proportion of time spent in any psychological, psychiatric, or mental hygiene center on the exhaustive psychological evaluation of the client or patient, it seems as though this *must* serve a useful purpose insofar as psychotherapy is concerned. Yet the more I have observed therapists, and the more closely I have studied research ... the more I am forced to the conclusion that such diagnostic knowledge is not essential to psychotherapy. It may even be that its defense as a necessary prelude to psychotherapy is simply a protective alternative to the admission that it is, for the most part, a colossal waste of time. There is only one useful purpose I have been able to observe which relates to psychotherapy. Some therapists cannot feel secure in the relationship with the client unless they possess such diagnostic knowledge. Without it they feel fearful of him, unable to be empathic, unable to experience unconditional regard, finding it necessary to put up a pretense in the relationship. (1957, s. 246)

The general and the unique

It is impossible not to categorize persons we meet. To make distinctions is our way of thinking. However, the more a person becomes known, the less he or she fits into preconceived categories. The ethos of relational therapy is to understand that the intersubjective meeting is unique.

Therapeutic understanding fluctuates between I and Thou and I and It (Buber, 1923). It is unrealistic that we should not sort patients into categories; humans always do. It would be naïve to believe that we do not categorize people just because we do not know use psychiatric diagnoses. Even if we are not familiar with the criteria for depression and obsessive-compulsive disorder, we recognize the types. To see somebody as "unique" is an epistemological and ethical challenge (Levinas, 1972).

Illness and responsibility – brain and mind

Mental life has its origin in the brain. But does the brain direct my thoughts, my intentions? If I decide to go to Berlin, is it my brain that decides? Without delving into philosophical questions about the free will, it is subjectively apparent that although my thoughts are born in the brain, it is not compatible with our view of human consciousness and conscience to give responsibility for my decisions to the synapses and transmitter substances. If I leave my wife because I have fallen in love with another woman, I could not blame the synapses.

In all societies, there have been negotiations about which behaviours the nervous system can be charged for, and which are the choices of free will. Does the person with schizophrenia have a choice to stop hallucinating? Can the person with ADHD decide to focus better? Can the depressed decide to think in more constructive ways? Trivially, behaviours can be seen as decided by the will but influenced by the framework the nervous system sets. But in the moment, in the concrete situation, we are faced with these issues as dilemmas. How much do I have to take from the person with ADHD? Is it impossible for my depressed partner to take care of the garbage?

Therapists should not be naïve about the limitations the brain sets. The scepticism about diagnoses should not lead to rudeness in the face of functional deficits. But it is important to stay in the intersubjective world with the patient, to decide that whatever the limits may be, the patient has his subjectivity.

Diagnosis as negotiation

Psychological treatment is collaboration more than most other treatments. In somatic care, the patient's task is to report how he feels and accept the treatment, whether it consists of surgery or taking a tablet. Psychic difficulties are a different matter. If I do not get out of bed for a week, my wife or my psychiatrist may wonder if I am depressed. But if I say that I just do not feel like getting up, they may have to accept it. Other signs may accumulate. I may show all the external signs of a depression: I have no appetite, I have anxiety in the morning, I do not finish what I started, I seem to lack energy. "You are probably depressed", the psychiatrist may say. But the question remains under negotiation. My own interpretation lasts a long way.

A telling example of the lack of validity in psychiatric assessments is the impossibility to predict suicide. If we compare with a tumour, a physician can, with reasonable certainty, predict that a certain type of tumour in a certain body environment will lead to the person's death. But even though we know a number of factors that increase the likelihood of suicide, we can never know which of our patients will kill himself.

Goal setting

In all treatment, the therapist needs to agree with the patient about what the treatment should be about. If the treatment has a clear focus on a defined problem, it may be easy to keep the target (Michalak & Holtforth, 2006). Research suggests that therapy works best if the therapist and patient agree upon a direction for the treatment and are clear about how to get there (Wampold & Imel, 2015). In short-term dynamic therapies, goal setting is usually seen as essential for success (Mann, 1973; Sifneos, 1979).

Symptom-focused treatments have aims like reduction of symptoms or dysfunctional behaviour. In relational treatment, a more appropriate concept is focus (Summers & Barber, 2011). The aim may be to get rid of a depression, but the focus is to handle conflicts with the parents better. Foci may be to regain hope (Frank & Frank, 1993), to learn from new experiences in social relations (Allison & Fonagy, 2016), to trust one's own agentic capacity (Bohart, 2000).

There are good arguments for explicit focus setting. The patient's motivation for treatment probably increases if the therapist and the patient agree on their target. The success of the treatment can be evaluated if the focus is clear. In the communication systems model (Allison & Fonagy, 2016), the therapist's presentation of a cogent model about how she understands the origins of the patient's problems and how to work with them is the core of therapy.

However, if the patient comes with more complicated problems, problems of different kinds, or problems that cannot easily be captured as a specific goal, the therapist and the patient will need to negotiate and renegotiate about the goal during the treatment. Although agreement on focus setting is certainly important, the challenge is to make the procedure therapeutically useful. In a study of three initial sessions of nine experienced therapists (Oddli, McLeod, Reichelt, & Rønnestad, 2014), two main themes emerged. One was deliberations about whether the patient found the sessions meaningful; the other was ambivalence about change. Rather than specifying explicit foci, therapist and patient tried to find ways of working together.

Often, a therapy takes directions that the therapist did not anticipate or plan. Sometimes it is easy to get back to the original issue, but not seldom the therapist realizes that the conversation has taken a turn that deepens the complexity of the problems or opens for more important questions than the ones they started out with. To find useful formulations for the emotional suffering is an important therapeutic task. Too many patients have left treatments because they never got the time to find words for their unique emotional struggles.

The patient's resources

During the assessment, the therapist may want to understand how the patient's relational difficulties impede him from managing complicated relationship problems in creative and constructive ways. Although formal assessment of relational competencies may seem superficial or rigid, it may be useful for the therapist's understanding. Sometimes it may also be useful in the dialogue with the patient. This is a list of relevant competencies and propensities:

- Mentalizing
- Attachment
- Affect awareness
- Confidentiality and shallowness
- Closeness and distance
- Independence and dependency

- Vulnerability
- Empathy and integrity
- Spontaneity and reflection
- Conflict management

Secret agenda?

Psychoanalytic treatment has been criticized for not being open about how the therapist conceptualizes the patient's problems. If the patient is assumed not to be aware of the roots of his problems and unwilling to approach them, the therapist's hypotheses about them are by definition hard to communicate to the patient. "My guess is that you did not only love your dad but sometimes you were quite disappointed with him, and at times you even despised him" may not be what the therapist at the first session tells the patient who idealizes his father.

In reality, all therapists probably have thoughts that will not be formulated in the first session but may have significance for the treatment.

The patient's knowledge

People know how to handle psychological problems. It is part of human nature to manage relational and emotional problems. But for different reasons, the capacity may be insufficient or limited. The patient's adaptive resources may be depleted, the social network falters, the needed communication among family and friends is lacking. Parents may worry exaggeratedly about their seemingly sad and passive children, people may feel compelled to behave in ritualistic ways, people get in conflict more often than they wish.

The problems are not always a mystery to them; they may have apparent relations to their life situations. Patients often know quite a lot about the causes of their problems, although they may close their eyes. They may have ideas about what might work and what they have already tried without success. Sometimes they also know what kind of therapist they need. If not, they quickly form an opinion. Even people who have not checked online who the therapist is or what kind of help may be most appropriate for them get an opinion at the first contact about how the person they meet can help them. In contrast to somatic healthcare, psychological treatment starts with explicit or implicit negotiations about how to understand the patient's problems and what to do about them.

The patient makes his assessment when he starts treatment. He tries to understand who the therapist is. He may wonder if she has worked for a long time, maybe so long that she has got tired of her work, if she will be able to understand how worried he feels, if she will look down on him for not daring to take conflicts, if he can tell her that he does not want to have sex without becoming ashamed, if she is married and has children, why she has a blouse and not a sweater. Assessments of the expert by the patient is common in all health care contacts. However, in psychotherapy, the patient's assessment of the therapist's credibility and competence is vital for the treatment process.

David

David was referred to his therapist Anne from a primary care doctor. From the referral, she knew that David was married and had children, that he was severely depressed, anxious, and probably drank too much. He had repeatedly been on sick leave and he had tried psychotropic medication of various kinds and psychological treatments without much success. She also knew that there was a notification to the social service about his behaviour with his children.

When they met for the first time, Anne read the referral to David. She asked him what he thought of his situation and what kind of help he thought he needed. David started talking about his fears of panic attacks. He thought his depression was a natural consequence of them.

He told Anne about his relationship with his wife and his children. He underlined that he loved them very much and that he was very anxious about his marriage.

He has grown up with a single mother. He thinks that has affected him a lot in relationships. In particular, he often feels lonely when he is with others. He is not visibly shy, and he does not know how much his sense of loneliness is noticeable. But it is hard for him to be in groups. Although he talks with others and they probably think he is nice and social, he often feels that he is on the outside.

Anne asked him to fill in some self-assessment forms. It turned out that David scored high on both the depression and anxiety forms. On a form about self-rated attachment style, he scored high on avoidant attachment style. And on a questionnaire about interpersonal problems, he had high scores on submission and conflict avoidance but also on impulsivity. On the alcohol form, he came under the threshold of abuse.

Anne perceived David as a kind person. She appreciated his low-keyed style and thought he was insightful about how his past relationships might have affected him. She told him that she thought the activation strategies that he tried in the previous treatment might have been helpful, but she realized that he was not motivated and that in the end, he had made them at his wife's urging. She appreciated that he made efforts to do things with his children.

They agreed during the first session that Anne would encourage him to maintain and develop his social contacts. She asked him to notice his feelings when he met persons, and to be curious about his reactions on occasions when he felt lonely. She proposed that they should try to understand how his life experiences had affected him and his problems. In particular, she thought it was significant that he had lost his father and that he apparently had longed for a replacement but also had become sceptical when his mother met some other man.

It seemed like a reasonable aim to help him get in touch with and to clarify feelings of loneliness and exclusion in his childhood to see how they disturbed him in his current relationships.

She summarized that they would have two foci, one targeting his current avoidance of social contacts and the other directed towards the consequences of feelings of abandonment and loneliness during childhood. In the diagnosis box in the medical record, she ticked that David had Major Depression and fulfilled some criteria of Generalized Anxiety and Panic attacks. Afterwards, she realized that they had not talked about alcohol problems or the notification to social authorities. She started wondering whether he was perhaps friendlier and more accommodating than she really felt adequate. Almost all the time, he agreed with her and thought her ideas were good. Anne reflected on how genuine his positive attitude really felt to her. If he continued in this way, she could become quite annoyed with him. It struck her that David never talked about anger or irritation although some relationships seemed to be quite stressful. She decided to talk with him about his potential irritation with Inga, the young woman at his work, and maybe also about the relationship with his uncle's family when he was a boy. As Anne thought it was important that he continue the activation attempts, even though he did not think he had any use of it, she thought it might be important to challenge him with this reasonable demand not only for the concrete gain of social contacts but also in order to test the relational dynamics between them.

At the next session she initiated a talk about his colleague:

– When you talk about Inga, I have thought about how I think I would have reacted if I were you. I guess I would get quite irritated on her at times. But you don't seem to.
– No, I think it's fine that she shows her knowledge, that's good for all of us.
– Sure, but you can come with knowledge in different ways. I get the impression that you feel she is overbearing sometimes.
– It's not that bad, it is fun for her that she can be proud of what she can.
– I guess you hear that I'm challenging you for acting with so much kindness.
– Yes you may be right that I'm too meek but that's how I feel.
– What do you think about feeling this way? And that I think you might be irritated?
– Well I can understand that you think I should be annoyed or something.
– And that I'm almost trying to punch you into the feeling?
– It's not that bad.

– Maybe not. But it strikes me that it feels a bit weird that first I get the impression that you should be angrier with Inga and now I feel almost annoyed that you are, let's say, so accommodating with me. Right now, it feels like you can't get annoyed. Whatever I say, you agree.
David looks down and seems to hesitate.

– My wife tells me all the time that I should put my foot down towards Inga. I just feel stupid and failed when I don't react the way people think I should. I think my wife doesn't respect my feelings.
Anne feels consternation. She has been categorical, and not very empathic. She had a hunch, but she put together her own puzzle without much curiosity about David.

– Let me think openly about this. I think you have reason to be angry, or at least irritated, not only at Inga but also in other situations. I guess I still think you might be angry at her. But you also tell me something else. You seem not to feel understood, and I guess you feel frustrated. Let's talk more about that feeling.

The therapist's purpose in this dialogue is to get a first sense of who David is and to test his interest in talking about his reflections about relationships, with Anne and with others, when she challenges him. It is not obvious that the therapist's reaction has much to do with what the patient comes to therapy for. The therapist explores her own reactions about what it is like to be with David by talking about her reactions. She also shows that she is curious about their interaction. The link to his problems is something that may come later. At this stage, the intention is to invite David to a dialogue about feelings that may be associated with the foci of the therapy.

How to do in practice

Relational therapy has an open view on goal setting and agreement on the therapeutic activities (Safran, 2002). This does not mean that goals should not be discussed. On the contrary, focused talk about where the patient is now and what he wants to attain is an evident aspect of the therapy process. Quite a few patients start therapy without a clear idea of how their suffering should be named or presented. If the therapist suggests how to understand the problems and how to work with them (Fonagy, Luyten, & Allison, 2015), the patient may negotiate these ideas and possibly take a stand in another direction.

The initial steps

When the patient initially comes to therapy, he usually brings his own formulations. The first task for the therapist is to frame the patient's history into formulations that make his problems treatable. Such (re)formulations take place in all talking therapies (Davis, 1986; Peräkylä, 2019). On the way to "making therapy", the patient needs some guidelines about how to proceed. Should he produce free associations and dreams, descriptions of problematic thoughts, problematic behaviour, or problematic relationships?

The basic tool for understanding the patient is the therapist's curiosity about the patient and her own reactions to what the patient presents. The therapist could ask herself questions like:

- How does the feeling I get for the patient match with his description about how other people seem to react to him, his problems, and difficulties?
- What am I surprised about in my reactions to the patient?
- What impression do I think he wants to make on me?
- Is this a person I want to know better?
- Is there anything that I immediately feel I ought to address but that I also feel is difficult to talk about?

In relational therapy, the focus will be on affects in relationships. What kind of emotions does the patient describe in recurring relational patterns? Is he curious about his own and others' motives, does he reflect on the feelings he shows, does he comment on feelings that the therapist may believe and perhaps suggest that he might feel, is he open about knowing the reasons why he acts as he does and why others act as they do.

The focus is also on the therapist's own feelings: does she feel worried about how the patient is with his children, is she cautious when she wants to say something about his mood, or does she get provoked? The countertransference is the therapist's barometer. Her emotional reactions contribute to her motivation to work with him, to get into a relationship with him. She needs to let them challenge her.

Often, the first impression is informative. The therapist may have talked with him on the phone before the call, or read a description, maybe a referral, about him. Despite this information, the actual meeting is usually surprising. The picture created in advance was in some respects true, in some not. Or it could be true in a way the therapist had not expected. Consider the situation when the patient comes because he has beaten his wife, more than once and with other persons as witnesses. What does the therapist expect? She creates a picture of such a person based on her own experiences of people, movies, or stories. How do her experiences in the session differ from her expectations?

It is important that the therapist makes efforts to be aware of her subtle reactions. Does the patient make it easy for her to understand him? Does he make a credible impression? Is she caught by his story? Does she have the feeling that he wants her to be caught by it? Does she feel he wants to impress her? Does she understand his way of reacting emotionally? Or is his way of describing what he has been through difficult to empathize with? In what way does he say things, with what rhythm, energy, melody, facial expression, and gesture? We make such assessments intuitively all the time, often without noticing them. In the initial conversations, it may be useful to monitor actively the impression that the patient gives.

Outside the therapy relationship

Although relational therapy is based on the idea that the relationship between the therapist and the patient creates important material for work, descriptions of relationships with other people are of great importance. One idea is to reflect on how others seem to react to the patient. What feelings and reactions does he seem to evoke in his wife, his children, his friends? It is a natural therapist reaction to "stand on the patient's side", to look at people in the patient's surroundings with the patient's eyes. It is the patient who gives pictures of them. His wife complains exaggeratedly, his boss puts unreasonable demands on him. Sometimes, we end up in believing that these descriptions are true and try to help the patient to find ways to respond to his creaking wife and demanding boss.

It may be of benefit to imagine what it might be like to be his wife or his boss. Are their reactions understandable, does the therapist recognize them in her own reactions? Do these reactions give her tips about what she might also feel? Maybe she is not alone in being critical. Using Racker's (1968) concepts, the therapist may need to make efforts to catch the complementary and not only the concordant countertransference.

A similar tool is to think about what it would be like to live with the patient. If the therapist met him every day, every morning, every night? What reactions does she surreptitiously sense might grow into big problems or strong feelings if she was constantly with him? Would she like to hug him, would she feel like a parent? Or would she feel disgusted by him?

The patient's reports about other persons' reactions may provide different kinds of information:

- They can provide a basis for the therapist to reflect about her own impressions of the patient in relation to how others respond to him. When she feels annoyed at the patient's tiresome way of describing his experiences and he says that he is disappointed that his wife often watches TV when he wants to talk with her about his problems, it gives her food for thought. It is not a truth; it is a chance for reflection.
- They provide a picture of the patient's tendency to place responsibility for difficulties on himself or others. Does he blame conflicts on his partner, or accuse himself of conflicts that arise? Is the therapist's first hunch that she should work on helping him see his own part in conflicts or should she rather help him realize that he is not responsible for all problems?
- They show if he describes emotions in a nuanced way and if he has an emotional register that includes many different kinds of emotions and emotions of different intensity.

- They give the therapist an opportunity to step into the patient's world, to create images of how the patient lives and what capacity he has to create stimulating and meaningful relations.

In sum, assessment in relational therapy is mutual, it is a first step on the road to formulate problems that are treatable in this therapeutic frame. The main task is to find ways to get involved in the patient's world.

12 Listen for your own thoughts, fantasies, and feelings

The tool

A basic tool in relational therapy is the therapist's attention to her own emotional reactions and fantasies about the patient, her counter-transference. The challenge for the therapist is to participate actively in the conversation and at the same time listen to her own emotional reactions to what the patient is saying and to what she herself is saying. This ability has been called *mindfulness-in-action* (Safran & Muran, 2000), meaning being consciously present, attentive, and non-judgemental in the ongoing interaction.

Talking to another person and at the same being aware of one's thoughts and feelings is not what we usually do. It does happen that we become acutely aware of what we think or feel when we talk with someone. But often we are not actively paying attention to it. Usually, minding about the on-going relationship is a fluctuating process as we intermittently realize what we feel or think. We are often at the "edge of awareness" (Preston, 2008), being aware of our feelings and fantasies for a while and then gliding back to the immediately ongoing interaction. Sometimes we identify a feeling during the conversation, and then, afterwards, discover another feeling that was also aroused but did not become conscious.

Therapists are used to work with the patient's emotions. To listen to what the patient says about what he feels about a particular situation, or what feeling he has at the current moment in the interaction, is standard therapy. Therapists may also wonder if the patient has unformulated, subconscious feelings, or if maybe one feeling is blocking another.

In relational therapy, the therapist uses the same approach to herself; she tries to become aware of what she is feeling herself. Sometimes she succeeds. But more often, she catches her feelings as esprits d'escalier, thoughts and feeling that are recognized when the patient has left. In supervision or during the evening walk, the therapist may realize what feelings were aroused in a dialogue with a patient. Training to become a better relational therapist means to move this attention and awareness as much as possible into the dialogue itself, into the moment, while being fully focused on the

DOI: 10.4324/9781003026914-12

conversation with the patient. But therapists also need to be overbearing with themselves, accepting lack or lacunae of emotional awareness.

The purpose

The purpose of attending to one's own reactions is twofold. First, they provide an understanding of how relationships that the patient creates with other persons may be felt. When the therapist has her own sense of what it is like to be with the patient, she can compare her reactions with how other people seem to respond to him. Does she get surprised by how others react, or does he recognize it in her own reactions? Second, reactions provide material for reflection, a basis for talking with the patient about the interaction. If she feels confused when she talks with him, she may be able to formulate it in order for them to reflect on it. Reflection on the interaction is best made when it happens. No feeling has such an obvious evidence as the one I sense right now. Sometimes, the perception of a feeling can be the basis for a conversation with the patient about it, sometimes it is enough that the therapist notices it and lets it contribute to her understanding of what it is like to be with the patient at this moment. Being aware of feelings does not mean that they must be communicated.

The dilemma

The therapist's reactions are born in the interaction with the patient. Some of them may be of a sort that most therapists would feel towards that particular patient (Winnicott, 1949). But how can we know? Most behaviour is ambiguous in its stimulus value. Haughtiness, to take an example, have many nuances and may evoke different reactions is different persons and situations. In addition, the reactions are the result of an interaction process: if the patient shows a certain kind of behaviour, it evokes a specific reaction in the therapist which, in turn, elicits a specific reaction in the patient. Soon into the interaction, the relationship is unique; what is evoked is created in a relationship that is subjective to the participants and perhaps far from what would have been elicited in with another therapist. The objective reaction has turned intersubjective.

It may seem strange that a patient comes to a therapist to hear about the therapist's personal reactions and feelings for him. It would seem more professional that the therapist conveys reactions that have some general validity. However, in a two-person perspective, reactions are seldom general. The dynamic between the notion that there is an objective counter-transference or projective identification with an unwitting therapist harboring what the patient disavows, and the idea that the therapist's re-actions to the patient are fundamentally influenced by both the therapist's and the patient's personalities, experiences and reaction patterns, and also by the interaction between them, is central to relational treatment. The tension is obvious between the notion that the work targets patient problems that exist outside the therapy room, at the same time as we realize that the feelings created, and used as material in the treatment, could have been completely different with someone else.

Principles

Our emotional reactions, our intuition, are basic to our survival and to our ability to understand social reality. It has strong genetic roots; we are often impressed by the sensitiveness of horses and dogs. Most of our intuition works out of awareness, automatically, without conscious reflection. Freud (1912a) suggested that the therapist should use his freely floating attention, having an open mind to her own reactions, in order to capture what the patient is conveying and especially that which does not have a clear verbal form. Reik (1949) wrote about the therapist's "third ear". The relational model of sensibility about affective communication is an extension of the interest in reading the nuances in interaction that is one of the pillars of psychoanalytic therapies.

Facilitative and explorative therapeutic stance

It may be useful to compare the relational therapeutic stance with the approach characterized by facilitative emotional presence advocated in the Rogerian humanistic tradition. Both, of course, have a strong focus on the therapist's sensitivity about the emotional interaction, the use of intuition, the therapist's curiousness about the subtle or hidden nuances in the conversation.

In Rogerian person-centred treatment, a listening and responsive approach is prescribed for the therapist. The therapist is empathic, genuine, and respectful towards the patient, showing emotional presence. Most therapists likely agree that this is a good professional and ethically correct approach to patients. However, from a relational perspective, the facilitative approach would not be enough. A significant possibility for relational work emerges when the therapist is incapable or unwilling to be empathic, genuine, and respectful. Openings for reflection and change grow in the empathic gaps.

What when the therapist is really tired of her patient feels scared of him, or gets turned on by him? The ground for the facilitative approach is the one-person model: the therapist's stance of emotional presence is the soil for the patient's explorations of his potential. The therapist approach is normative: it is the therapist's responsibility to retain the facilitative stance. In contrast, the relational entry is curiousness about countertransference, about tiredness, fear, or arousal. The overarching approach is to facilitate the patient's movement, but the immediate reaction to negative feelings is inquisitiveness.

Subtle signals

It may be hard to capture subtle indications of emotional reactions. Gendlin (1996) argued that patients who have the ability to focus on and make themselves aware of vague and unclear, often bodily, sensations, which can subsequently be formulated as experiences, thoughts and feelings, have the capacity to use psychotherapy. People experience the outside world with their entire bodies before understanding it in a conceptual sense. Gendlin used the word "focusing" to describe engaged accepting attention, leading to a "felt sense". He described this characteristic in patients, but the same attention process is important for therapists.

Inspired by Bion's (1967) concept of reverie, Ogden (1994b) explored how fantasies, whims, stray thoughts may be clues that emerge in the therapist and eventually will turn out to be related to the patient's problems. "The most mundane, everyday aspects of the background workings of the mind (which appear to be completely unrelated to the patient), and other forms of bodily sensations and body related fantasies" can be important indications of intuitively captured interactional processes (Ogden, 1994a, pp. 4–5).

Being emotionally accessible to the patient is a prerequisite for psychological treatment. This means in a general sense that the therapist is responsive, accepting, tolerant, and interested in the patient. The more specific psychoanalytic meaning of the concept of emotional availability is tied to the concept projective identification. This concept focuses on how the therapist may be "used" by the patient (Ogden, 1989). In the projective identification process, the patient behaves in, often indiscernible, ways that evoke specific reactions in the therapist (Bion, 1962; Ogden 1989). A typical example is the therapist who feels sad after talking with a patient who disavows his own sadness.

In the relational perspective, the therapist's reactions are no blueprints of the patient's unrecognized feelings but rather indications of the emotional atmosphere in the interaction. The therapist offers her emotional reactions, an amalgam of her own habitual reactions and her situationally evoked feelings, and responses to the patient's emotional position. It is never admissible to make the patient responsible for the therapist's feelings. But it is always admissible to try to be as attentive as possible to the reactions that the interaction with the patients evokes.

David

David had agreed with Anne that he would take a rather long walk every day. He should walk for up to an hour.

- It was great that you walked. Were you tired?
- Well, I can't say I was tired, although I walked for a while.
- How far did you go?

- I went up to the grocery store and then I walked back through the park.
- It is a bit, but it's not that far.

Anne knew about the surroundings and wondered if it really takes an hour to walk that round from David's house. She would guess that it takes a maximum of half an hour. Although she feels satisfied that David has taken the walk, she is also disappointed that it was actually a fairly short round. She chooses not to say anything about what she feels because she wants the feelings to become clearer to her. Instead, she asks a little more about how it felt to him.

- How did you feel about doing it?
- In a way it was ok, but it was a bit strange, too. It feels odd to practice walking.
- Do you want us to decide that you also take some social contacts during the walk until the next session? Just take a coffee with someone.
- I don't know. I don't feel like doing things just for the sake of it.

Anne feels a little bit annoyed at David's dismissive attitude to her suggestions. She senses that he pretends not to understand the points with them. But she chooses not to say anything about this either.

- So how do you want to get more stimulation?
- Do I need stimulation? I do things with the kids sometimes. Isn't that enough? Maybe I could be allowed to rest when I'm on sick leave? It seems that all therapists have been taught that patients have to do things when they are depressed. Is there any evidence that it works?

Anne realizes that a conflict is approaching. She is unclear about what she really feels about it. Does she get annoyed at David for being reluctant and that he is now slightly aggressive? Or is she worried about how the conflict between them will develop? She feels uncertain but chooses to try to comment on how she views the situation.

- It seems we have kind of a conflict coming up. My feeling is that you think these activity programs are stupid and I have no desire to nag you about them. I think I would also feel stupid if someone said I should take walks just for the sake of it. Do I hear right if I think you're annoyed with me also?
- Yes, and it's no wonder. I've tried this before and it didn't help. I thought I'd get some other help from you.

Anne now feels openly criticized. She starts to think about what she has ended up in. Although it is fine if depressed people activate themselves, she knows that David at least partly has come to her because he did not think there was any point with these activation programs.

- You may be right that it does not make any sense to walk, especially as I know you do things anyway. But I do feel annoyed that you didn't say it in advance. It is pretty pointless that we agree on things that you do not really want to do.

Anna realizes that she sounds irritated. David becomes quiet and looks out the window. Anne wonders if he was hurt. Should she perhaps be more understanding? But she thinks she doesn't want to give up, she can't just feel pity for him. She waits for some seconds.

‒ I was thinking about my reaction. I guess you felt that I became a bit pushy about your walks. I have that tendency. And when you expressed your discontent, I became a bit worried. So now there are two feelings in me: go ahead and Be careful. Any ideas about that?

   Anne entered this dialogue with an annoyance on David. She is now in a more complex emotional state where, in addition to the irritation, she also feels a little ashamed, and also more understanding of David. She waited a while to say what she felt but eventually did so and then got into a conversation that to some extent changed the emotional tone between them. She now presents her feelings as material for reflection, inviting David to reflect on their interaction.

How to do in practice

The essence of this tool is to practice the art of being unguarded in relation to one's own inner life, feelings, and ideas. The therapist tries to be aware of her reactions, to be curious and non-evaluatively present when experiencing them. To be mindful.

In everyday interactions with others, we use our implicit mentalizing to handle interactions. This is the lube oil for effective human interaction. Reactions come in various shapes, overwhelming and clear or hardly detectable, mentally or bodily, as fantasies or as self-evident and non-disputable reactions. They are there all the time but usually not in focus.

We are often perplexed when asked on the spot what we feel. We handle interactions but we are often without words for what happens emotionally. Every supervisor who has asked the supervisee what she felt in an interactional moment with a patient has met the answer: "Well, I felt that he found it difficult to". Although, if asked, we would most of the time agree that we are in a specific emotional state, the exact wording of this state is often a challenge.

In interaction with others, we are emotional all the time; it is part of implicit relational knowing. We can practise becoming aware of it by, for instance, actively trying to capture our feelings and thoughts when we are with known or unknown people. Or when we read books or watch a movie.

It requires both mental discipline and sensitivity to work with this kind of mental curiosity. It takes some scrutiny to capture the mood of a relationship. When the interaction has been going on for a while, we often are like fish in the water; we know nothing other than what we are in. The fish may discover how obvious the water was when it was landed. What is the equivalent for us? Some suggestions:

Notice your reactions

• Right at the beginning of the relationship, when you are not yet in wheel tracks

- When something unexpected happens (criticism, interruption, joy)
- When you feel confident that something must be said or absolutely cannot be said

Recurrent or emergent?

The issue of the whether countertransference reactions are predictable, recurrent in the patient's relationship, or emergent, co-created, is crucial to the usefulness of the therapist's reactions. Mitchell (2000) discussed different ways of understanding relational patterns. He argued that both the recurrence and the emergence perspective are valid and useful. There is, certainly, an empirical question about the extent of repetition of evocative patterns. But it is also a question of usefulness. Is it meaningful to insist that the therapist's reaction is similar to others' reactions or is there more therapeutic value in opening for reflection on the therapist's specific reaction, without knowing how general it might be? In practice, the relational point is that the therapist's unique emotional reaction has an affective impact that is more obvious that an argument about its ubiquitousness.

An example:

The patient talks about how valuable it is to come and talk about his concerns. He does not think the therapist has to make much effort to come up with reflections or solutions because he can actually find them himself if he only has someone to talk with. The therapist is somewhat frustrated and thinks that the patient might as well talk with his wife about this. She feels that her expert knowledge will not be of any use if therapy is to listen to how the patient comes up with his ideas and solves his problems on his own. Successively, she understands that the patient has a similar way of being with others; he loves to describe how he takes care of himself. In his view, other persons admire his abilities. The therapist gets the impression that other persons also may become frustrated by the patient's self-sufficiency.

One way to handle the situation would be for the therapist to listen for reactions from others. The patient might suggest that although his wife or his parents try to help him, he is his own best helper, thus opening for an interpretation that the patient might look down on the therapist too. Or the patient might describe situations where people have forced their help on him, thus suggesting that he may have a strong need for autonomy. These are attempts to put the pieces together in a jigsaw puzzle about how to *understand* his behaviour. In relational treatment, it may unfold like this:

The therapist feels a little bit nervous.

- I've been trying to catch how I feel about my impression that you always seem have your own solutions to your problems. It doesn't feel like I'm doing any good for you.

- I think it's great that I can formulate my thoughts with you, that helps me to think better.

(The therapist feels a little annoyed that the patient does not seem to understand what she is after.)

- Do you have any idea how it might feel to me?
- It sounds like you are not satisfied, but you should know that you ask great questions that make me think better.

(The therapist is still annoyed but also a bit surprised.)

- It's an interesting and also somewhat curious situation. I think you have the right to get more help from me, but you think what I do is ok. For me, it feels like I don't really know if I'm doing any good. What do you think of that?
- I wonder if you're trying to give me guilt feelings for not listening to your good advice.

(The therapist thinks the conversation becomes awkward, but she also gets more energy.)

- Well, I don't know ... that's not what I think, but we might try to understand how it is. I'm the one who make difficulties, you seem to be satisfied. In some way I guess I have the feeling that you try to control what I'm saying.
- You can't say that I control how we talk. You may pick up whatever you want. But I understand that you have an idea of how this should be going. I should come up with a problem and then you'll give me a suggestion on what to do about it or how to think about it. I don't think it's a good way to work. It must be better if I have ideas myself.

The conversation continues with an exploration of the feelings evoked by the conflict between the therapist's desire to contribute and the patient's desire to come up with his own ideas. The patient feels criticized and the therapist feels awkward for initiating a conflict. She loses the clarity in her understanding and feels a little lost. The situation has become more complex. The initial question about understanding the reasons for the patient's wish to find solutions himself has been put to the side; instead, issues about initiative and autonomy have come to the fore. Instead of insisting on understanding the patient's need for control, the therapist opens for feelings of bewilderment.

By intervening with an immediacy self-disclosure, a conflict is evoked between patient and therapist. The conversation has another emotional colour than it had when the talk started. In contrast to the experience of reading a book, when the reader's feelings only develop from the impressions of the text, the therapist actively intervenes and becomes influenced by the following process. If the therapist had been quiet, she could have escaped this somewhat uncomfortable situation. Now, she has created material to work with.

Feelings are not interpretations

It often takes effort to find one's feelings, they may be "unbearably light" also for the therapist. Therapists often feel bewildered when asked what they feel: "Well I felt that he was really angry at his wife, but he didn't allow himself to show it". To capture one's own feelings is different from interpreting. A therapist may think that a depressed girl tries to look charming because she needs to keep away her sad and angry feelings. The therapist's feelings may be delight or worry. Guessing about hidden feelings is something else. Although they may come simultaneously, it is important for therapists to stay in their immediate experience.

13 Stay in the present, be concrete and specific

The tool

Life is in the present moment. The meaningful emotional experience is in the ongoing interaction, in the perceived immediacy of stories from the past and dreams we weave for the future. Vital experience is not general, it is not "in principle", it is concrete and specific.

In order to promote therapeutic presence, it is important to encourage the patient to be as detailed as possible in his descriptions, and for the therapist to be as detailed as possible in her descriptions of what is happening between herself and the patient.

Therapeutic presence thus has two aspects. One is to invite concreteness in the patient's narratives and descriptions. A film cannot be abstract, neither can a dream. Emotional experiences are associated with images, sounds, concrete narrated words. To be present in the intersubjective experience of the patient's world, the therapist needs to encourage concreteness. To take part in the patient's stories, the therapist must know how the people in them look, what tone of voice they have, what they perceive of each other, and what emotions are aroused in them. An analogy might be to think about how it is to read a novel. An indication that the reader has come into the book is that she sees the scenes in the book in her mind. If no concrete scenes emerge, she will lose interest. If the details in the patient's story do not appear in the therapist's head, the story is not concrete enough.

The other aspect concerns presence in the therapeutic interaction. Psychological treatment is, at best, an engaged exchange where the participants, with their feelings, desires, and fantasies, deal with issues and problems that are important to the patient and that become important to the therapist. This requires a curiosity about what happens in interaction with the patient, verbally and beside the words. Experiences in a relationship are easily perishable; they are most clearly alive in the present moment. Often, we do not know what we feel or think, what the story we hear is about, what happens between us. An important part of the therapeutic work is to find out.

DOI: 10.4324/9781003026914-13

The purpose

Details make experiences understandable. By attending to them we understand emotions in stories. When we hear the nuances and details in a story, we get into it. In the detailed descriptions, both the patient's and our own, of what happens between us, we can, to be sure, lose foothold. Most human problems are multifaceted and complicated. If they were simple, the solution would be simple, and the patient could get help from someone else. The challenge for the therapist is to see the complications, to understand, even if the patient at first does not, why he came to us and not to his friend. And to avoid the simple solutions that friends can come up with. We must dare to let the complexity hit us, try to find the place where the patient got lost. The more complicated the impasse, the closer we are to the patient's actual situation.

The dilemma

A movie or a book starts with a concrete scene. The scene serves as entrance to the larger drama, the life context that we will eventually get to know. If we only see the first scene and nothing more, we cannot know how representative it is for the larger context. But if the book only offered a description of a context, we would not be caught. It is the immediacy, the details that awaken our emotions and imaginations. In relational treatment, we search for the concrete. The whole picture comes successively.

After a session, the therapist may realize that the scene that took hold of her was not an ordinary scene in the patient's life. Sometimes the patient becomes annoyed that the therapist gets stuck in a situation that the patient does not perceive as important. The tension between the detail and the overall view may come in conflict. That is natural and unavoidable. If the therapist's fixation to a situation irritates the patient, the therapeutic situation has evolved to a potentially meaningful conflict – and to a possibility to present other concrete situations.

Principles

It is not specific to relational therapy that the therapist wants a detailed picture of the patient's problems and of his life situation. In emotion focused therapy, the therapist wants to get a detailed account of the patient's emotional reactions, in which situations they are aroused, what the emotions are about, what they are directed towards. If a patient is depressed, a cognitive therapist may want to know what thoughts are associated with the depressive symptoms and in which situations. All therapy is based on detailed analyses of problems.

Relational therapy focuses on the emotional interaction in the treatment relationship. Emotional interaction does not arise by itself. It occurs when the patient talks about situations that catch the therapist's curiousness. Or when he does not, and the therapist becomes curious about that. The more images she gets from the patient's life, the more emotions are aroused in her. More emotional interaction in the relationship gives more chances.

An illustration:

The patient is often busy solving problems for others, providing solutions for others. When the therapist has a cold, he gives advice on how to get well; when the therapist discloses that she is going on vacation to Greece, he comes with information brochures about Greece that he happened to find on the way. The therapist gets tired of all the good advice.

The therapist has the options to ask the patient about his reasons and feelings about his behaviour and to disclose her own reaction.

– I have thought about your helpfulness. I'd like to say something about my reactions. Although I do appreciate your kindness, I would like to share a reaction that I had when you gave me the brochure. It was divided. As I said, I thought it was nice. But I also realized that I got a bit irritated, feeling somewhat invaded by your helpfulness. I don't know really how to explain, but it was like you tried to get more into my life than I want to.
– I must assure you that I have no intention of meddling in your life.
– *The patient looks ashamed. The shame reaction was not what the therapist had hoped for.*
– I get the feeling that you get ashamed.
– Well, it's no problem, I just happened to see the brochures.
– I am looking for the feeling. I realize you want to be kind. Do you have any other feeling?
– Of course, I feel a bit sad about your reaction.
– Would you call it hurt?
– Not really, I'd rather say that I may be naïve about others' reactions. I guess I feel stupid.

The therapist tries to chisel out the specific affective reaction. Using Stern's words, the therapist takes a small step to develop "unique and evolving understandings and forms of relational engagement that we co-create with our patients in response to their uniquely complex psychological organizations and therapeutic needs, both in the immediate analytic moment and cumulatively over time" (Stern, 2017, p. 95).

The fragment and the whole

A movie often starts with a very specific and narrow picture of an event. We may see a family having breakfast, follow their conversation, and successively create a picture of who they are and what relationships they have with each other. The director offers a small part of the people's life world. When we have seen the entire film and think back to the first scene, we realize that it only gave one of several possible perspectives, an angle on the lives of the characters. We may even think that the director deliberately wanted to deceive us, creating a picture that she could then turn around in the film kaleidoscope.

When we try to get a description of a person's relationships, we sometimes focus on details that do not give a "true" picture of the person's whole world. The feelings aroused in us from the patient's story are created by the descriptions he happened or wanted to give us. Other descriptions, other stories would arouse other feelings.

So we end up with a dilemma: if we want a complete picture of the patient's world, we cannot get all the details and then the description will lack must and colour. If, on the other hand, we want to get the details that create feelings in us, we always get a skewed and incomplete perspective. Blake's poem about seeing the world in a grain of sand and the sky in a flower suggests that the part captures the essence of the whole. In a poetic sense, it is true. But we do not know and should not assume it.

People live in stories and images. We understand ourselves and others through them. Sometimes the story is a verbal description that goes from one point to another. Sometimes an image makes the same emotional impact. The picture of the dead Alan on the beach on the Mediterranean was as effective as a story to awaken our feelings and fantasies about the hardships of refugees. The emotions evoked by stories and images are the material that we use in therapy.

David

David has quarreled with his mother. He is by nature a cautious man and they do not quarrel often. When he becomes angry at her, he tries to calm himself because he is afraid that he will hurt her. Sometimes, he has tried to talk with her about how he felt when he was a boy. He wonders why she did not try to get another job so she could be at home in the evenings. When he brings up such things with her, she gets irritated and starts defending herself. David does not get anything out of it. When he last visited her, she had started sorting out old photos. With the photos on the table, they talked about his childhood. He asked why the relationship with Peter ended. She became angry and said that she did not want to talk with him about that. She wanted to have her secrets. She knew that David liked him, but he couldn't see the whole picture, she said. David became angry at her and told her that he was in his right to know what happened. Anne thinks she can see the situation in her mind.

–   It seems to be quite a special situation. She has her life in front of her on the table and you try to talk about shared painful memories. What did she look like?

- I don't know. I didn't look at her, I was shy in some way.
- But you looked at the photos?
- When I came, I think she became embarrassed and tried to hide some of them. I thought I'd ask her about the photos she put aside but I didn't dare. I think they were pictures of her with other men.
- I guess you may have felt consternated.
- Shameful, but also irritated. I'm tired of this sensitivity about my childhood.
- Did you tell her?
- All the time I'm in this mixture of feelings. I guess you think I should have talked with her about it. You don't know how she looks at these occasions.
- How does she look?

Anne continues asking him about the details as the narration evokes affects both in David and in herself. She wants to get the detailed picture; she wants to see it before her eyes.

How to do in practice

Therapeutic presence

Presence can be described as "being aware of and centred in oneself while maintaining attunement to and engagement with another person" (Hayes & Vinca, 2017, pp. 86–87). Being present, with emotions and thoughts, imagination and empathy, is important in all constructive meetings between people. By the end of his life, Rogers reflected that his approach could be summed up to one principle: that the therapist should be fully present with the patient. "I am inclined to think that in my writing I have stressed too much the three basic conditions. Perhaps it is something around the edges of those conditions that is really the most important element of therapy – when my self is very clearly, obviously present" (Rogers in interview with Baldwin, 2000, s. 30).

Emotional presence, meaning the therapist's deliberate stand as much as the evoked atmosphere in the relationship, is a defining aspect of the therapeutic interaction that characterizes relational therapy (Gendlin, 1996; Stern, 2004a). Many interventions can contribute to a stronger sense of presence. When the therapist meticulously asks for details in the patient's story, she comes closer to the patient's lived experience. When she suggests a feeling that the patient may have had, she may get closer to the patient's mind.

The relational dialectics also open for other therapist experiences. In her striving to remain present, to listen with an open mind, to pay attention to how the relationship develops, the therapist often fails. She may lose her concentration, start thinking about something else. Or she may get stuck in something the patient said a while ago.

She thinks the patient looked sad. She wonders if she was right, she asks herself if she can say it. She loses her focus; the ongoing interaction is not quite in her attention. Presence is not a state where the therapist can park herself, it evolves and wanes.

Presence is to strive to be present in the actual interaction, and to be present in the observation of the mind's ramblings. The therapist, to be sure, tries to retain an evenly suspended attention (Freud, 1912a), to listen with her third ear (Reik, 1949). But she is also attentive when presence weakens. It is often difficult to "listen in the effortless way" (Reich, 1951, p. 25).

In clinical practice, the distinction between the humanistic exhortation on presence (Geller & Greenberg, 2012) and the relational curiosity about its waxing and waning (Ogden, 1994a) may be marginal. In principle, however, the humanistic stance focuses on the patient, whereas the relational position is curiosity on the fluctuations of presence in the interaction.

Therapeutic presence and mindfulness

Mindfulness meditation is recommended in many therapy forms as an effective technique for various problems. The patient practising mindfulness meditation may get a mental distance to stressful and emotionally disturbing thoughts.

Therapeutic presence has similarities with mindfulness meditation. The aim of mindfulness is to be present in the actual experience without getting caught in it (Santorelli, 1999). Mindfulness implies concentration on perceptions and thoughts. Safran and Muran (2000) used the concept mindfulness-in-action, meaning a non-judgemental awareness of the therapeutic interaction.

Mindfulness as an observational and non-judgemental technique fits well into the psychoanalytic stance, for patient as well as for therapist. However, in contrast to mindfulness meditation as a method for the individual, the psychoanalytic perspective is relational (Safran & Reading, 2008, p. 124), the focus is on the interaction. Ivey (2015) describes the relational stance as mindfulness-inclusive instead of mindfulness-based. The focus is on new experiences in the therapeutic relationship rather than insights into the contents and functions of the patient's mind (Ivey, 2015, p. 388; Sugarman, 2006).

> It is not enough to see [the therapeutic] relationship as ground for technique or as reflection of personal dynamics, but the potential for change is maximized by the recognition of relational experience as it unfolds. (Muran, 2019, p. 9)

From I – Thou to I – it

It is often easy for therapists to jump to assessments and categorizations, to put the patient in a box. For some, diagnoses may be the most natural choice. "He shows signs of autism". For others, concepts like mentalizing deficits and insecure attachment are more appealing.

Categorizations imply that a frame of interpretation is put around the concrete story. When the therapist thinks she realizes that what she hears belongs to the category "partner violence" or "childhood sexual abuse", some doors seem to open, and others to become less visible. The patient also puts interpretative frames around his experiences. "I think I have ADHD" or "My mom said that I'm introvert like she".

People need to interpret and categorize, themselves, others, and experiences. It is a challenge for the therapist to help the patient, and herself, to break up, challenge her own and the patient's general descriptions, to avoid the tendency to see "it" (Buber) or "das man" (Heidegger) instead of Thou.

Presence and other mental states

No therapy school has more than psychoanalysis contributed to the idea that the therapist should see behind the surface, find hidden secrets. And no other school has more clearly pointed to the usefulness in focusing on the patient's ongoing experiences in the transference. The great challenge for the relational therapist is to redirect the urging to find hidden meanings and stay with the emotionally present.

Being in the present is not an activity, it is a mental stance. There is nothing as simple as saying that therapy is about being in the here-and-now and nothing as difficult to do. It is not that difficult to close the eyes and pay attention to the breathing. But to be in the present while interacting with another person is not always easy. Desires, expectations, assessments, and tactical considerations stand in the way. "I have to try to make her understand that she is angry, but she always tries to be kind and accommodating". "If I start talking about her dad she will start crying and I don't know if that takes the treatment ahead". We calculate, assess, and analyze. It is, in a sense, natural, because that is what we do in regular conversations. Intellectualizing is too easy, the hard task is to remain in the present.

14 Be spontaneous, be genuine, and talk about your reactions

The tool

Psychological treatment should be based on scientific knowledge. Words like technique, systematic method, replicability, and planned intervention fit into that view. Relational treatment is also based on scientific principles. Certain methods and techniques are appropriate for relational therapy, they define the frames and the direction of the work. They have been found to be effective in systematic studies or repeatedly in case reports. But in the session, the "living word", the "genuine gesture" are the tools. The art of relational therapy is to combine planning with spontaneity, well-balanced formulations with authenticity. Experience-near dialogue is important, what the therapist says should not "owe ... their inescapable quality to their conformity with the analyst's theory" (Stern, 2013b, p. 631). The therapist's stance is to be as responsive, and as emotionally present as she can.

And to be mindful about occasions when she is not. Aside from rudeness and lack of respect, the therapist cannot say anything wrong in relational treatment that cannot be amended and repaired. When things go wrong, the chance appears to reflect on what happened, to get hold of the evoked emotions, to reflect on differences in perspective and sensibility – to focus on the relationship.

The purpose

Genuineness is a facilitative therapist stance in the Rogerian view of psychotherapy. It is an obvious way to strengthen the alliance by showing the patient that the therapist is engaged in the interaction. This is an interventionist, one-person perspective. Another purpose of being genuine and spontaneous is to contribute to the creation of vital interaction. If the dialogue is engaged, emotionally saturated, characterized by curiosity, the therapist becomes part of the co-created mental world, opening for the evolvement of interactional patterns that can be explored (BCPSG, 2010). In this two-person perspective, the therapist makes herself available for unexpected processes between herself and the patient. By loosening the

DOI: 10.4324/9781003026914-14

therapeutic reins, the therapist exposes herself to interplay that is not predictable. On the superficial level, such spontaneity contributes to interpersonal events that can be reflected on. On a deeper level, it implies availability for implicit influence from the patient and the interaction, unforeseeable reactions, for becoming part of and sharing the patient's mental world.

The dilemma

You cannot interact alone, as little as you can waltz alone. Everyone who has waltzed knows that it is not just one who dances. A good dancer can lift a mediocre partner, a bad dancer can make it difficult for any dance cavalier. The pace certainly shows whether it is waltz or foxtrot. And there are some rules for how the waltz should be danced. But dancing really depends on the dancers. It depends on the experiences of both and on their joint effort. All mediocre dancers have danced with a partner who was perhaps also half-bad but where it was still thrilling. The dance is the third, inviting us to interact with it.

When we talk with each other, there are also rules. We know what is possible and appropriate to say. But the conversation gets life if it is open to new and unexpected initiatives (Black, 2003). Therapists have their favourites. If the patient is depressed and the therapist's view is that his social network is too small, she may try to persuade him to make more friends. If she thinks he is depressed because his mother left him when he was a child, she may try to help him get in touch with feelings about this. Or she may feel for comforting, advising, and motivating. She will do it her way, with her experiences and values, her style, her hopes, all the time hopefully influenced by the patient's responses. Spontaneity is always personal, although in good therapy appropriate for the patient.

Principles

Interaction is mutual. It is giving and taking, to try ideas and to see how the other responds. Sometimes, it is helpful for the patient to get recommendations and advice. A therapist has met quite a few patients with emotional and relational concerns, and it would be odd if she did not have some experience and knowledge to share with her patients. The advice is not an intervention, it is an aspect of being together in therapy.

The important question is not what to say, it is to attend to what happens when the therapist has given the interpretation, advice, the admonition, the suggestion, and to be curious about it. How does the patient react?

The therapist's authority

During her working hours, the therapist meets patients who not rarely consider her to be wise and helpful. Coming home, the family is not always so certain about the wisdom of their therapist wife and mother. Instead, the therapist may be confronted about shortcomings and unresolved conflicts. She becomes involved and embroiled in complex and sometimes seemingly unsolvable conflicts. In that life, she is no expert on hassles in relationships. It would be presumptuous and hopefully met with laughter if she put on an authoritative face and insisted that she is in fact trained in psychological treatment. We are quite satisfied that this is so. Friends who try to be therapists in their leisure time may be unbearable.

In one-person models of psychotherapy, it is possible to make a distinction between a professional and a personal self, in principle. The mental distance to the patient's problems makes it possible to retain an idea of external expertise. In relational therapy, however, the problems to be focused on are primarily those that arise in the interaction. We allow ourselves to be drawn into enactments more or less intentionally, getting ensnared in complicated relationships with the patient at the same time as we are experts who try to understand what is happening. When the therapist becomes spontaneous, really is in the relationship, the disciplining of a boundary between professional and personal becomes challenging. And there is no solution, just attempts to be aware of the dilemma.

To feel uncertain

It is understandable that therapists want guidelines about what to say in therapy. Treatment guidelines are welcomed by many therapists, there are even in some countries recommendations that psychological treatments should be manual based.

In reality, therapists are from time to time flummoxed, insecure, and doubtful (De Peyer, 2016; Slochower, 2017). An important aspect of the therapeutic stance is to stand vulnerability in the presence of the patient. The therapist needs confidence in the process more than in her ability. She has to use opportunities in the conversation to create understanding and find alternative options. It takes a process to arrive at such understanding; the process is the treatment.

One aspect of how the therapist should talk to the patient is to attempt to evaluate the patient's ability to use the therapist's intervention. There is extensive literature on how to assess the appropriateness of using confrontations or challenges. A traditional psychoanalytic view is that patients with low ego strength, low self-esteem should not get transference interpretations. Interestingly, the only randomized empirical study of this hypothesis (Høglend et al., 2008) found that patients with lower relational efficacy had more benefit from transference interpretations than patients with more relational ability.

An example:

The patient's siblings have broken their contact with him. His daughter says that if he separates from her mother, she will never have any contact with him. In the initial sessions, he seems to be desperate about his lone-liness. The therapist has the feeling that she does not contact him emo-tionally, she thinks he is just babbling. She thinks it is odd that he does not know why his siblings, whom he says he longs for, do not want to con-tact him.

–   I wonder why you don't know why your siblings won't talk with you.
–   I really don't know myself either.
    The therapist thinks this cannot be true. He must have some idea about it. It feels as if he closes the door in her face.
–   I realize it's a complicated situation, but I feel skeptical that you tell me the whole truth when you say you don't know.
–   So, you don't believe me? What's the point of talking with you if you don't believe me?
    The therapist feared this might happen but feels adamant to go on.
–   I get it that you can become angry, but I still wonder if you want to keep me in uncertainty. I'm thinking about what we're into. You may see me as confrontational, but from my side I just want to know more about you.
    Pause
–   I don't feel very comfortable about letting people know too much about me.

In the remainder of the session, they talk about the clash between the therapist's curiosity and the patient's cautiousness. At the next session, the patient is hesitant to continue the therapy. After some work, the patient can find words for his tendency to escape from emotionally complicated situa-tions. He realizes that this may be one reason for his family's distance to him.

Spontaneity as action

To be spontaneous may also be to act. Psychoanalytic therapy is known for firm limits on the therapist's actions; relational therapy has put an honor in breaking them. Examples may be flexibility about session frames, involve-ment with other persons, accepting gifts. There may be different reasons for acting. One is curiosity; to explore reactions that come up when the inter-action breaks rules. Breaking rules by principle is pointless, breaking them when needed may be decisive. The therapist who gives his private number to the patient shows consideration in a way that the patient realizes may be special (Sandberg, Gustafsson, & Holmqvist, 2017).

The therapist's self-disclosing

The therapist's self-disclosing is a specific form of openness. Self-disclosures and attention to the interaction that follows is key to relational therapy.

Spezzano (1998) even asked what "relational analysts do in between en-actments and self-disclosures".

There is a large literature on the reasons for self-disclosing and their usefulness (Alfi-Yogev, Hasson-Ohayon, Lazarus, Ziv-Beiman, & Atzil-Slonim, 2020; Hill & Knox, 2002; McCarthy & Betz, 1978). Self-disclosures can be of different kinds:

- Intentional communications about the therapist's life experiences.
- Intentional communication about the therapist's feelings and fantasies in the ongoing therapeutic interplay ("immediacy").
- Unintentional or unplanned information about the therapist like comments that can be interpreted in a way the therapist was not aware of, bur also clothing and furniture, tone of voice, mimics, gestures, ways of breathing.

The first category contains information about the therapist that is usually uncontroversial. Sometimes, therapists think the cooperation with the patient might be helped by her saying something about herself. Self-disclosing may in general promote equality in the therapeutic relationship (Mark, 2018). If used with discretion, it may be helpful (Hill, Knox, & Pinto-Coelho, 2018). A simple illustration:

The therapist wants to help the patient expose himself to social situations like entering the coffee room at work. The therapist has had a tendency to social anxiety and tells the patient about it. The patient may feel less ashamed and more encouraged to try.

Immediacy interventions are focused on the therapeutic here-and-now relationship, usually including the therapist's reactions (Hill, 2004; Kuutmann & Hilsenroth, 2012). The intention may to create material for mutual reflection (Mayotte-Blum et al., 2012). Immediacy disclosures can be seen as two-person versions of transference interpretations (DeFife, Hilsenroth, & Kuutmann, 2015).

If the therapist thinks she understands what is going on, self-disclosure may be an invitation to reflection on aspects of the interaction that the therapist finds important. The therapist may try to break an impasse, to invite to a third perspective on the interaction (Aron, 2006). Self-disclosing about the interplay may be helpful if they are made with sensitivity about the current need of the patient, and with detailed probing of the patient's reaction (Aron, 2006).

It may be hard for the therapist to decide when to talk about her own reactions. A metaphor could be that the patient arranges the stage for the presentation of his current problems, memories, or fantasies. The therapist waits until the stage is organized, the protagonists are presented. When something in the patent's play arouses feelings in the therapist, it may be time to talk.

Idealized spontaneity?

The openness and spontaneity that is a significant aspect of the relational method has been criticized on different grounds. An apparent risk is that the therapist idealizes her own personal reactions, believing that her counter-transference is the key to the patient's problems. Therapists may self-indulge in talking about their own reactions in a way that may be to the detriment of the patient (Slochower, 2017). Greenberg (2001) warned for a personality cult, Bernstein (1999) wrote about therapists being enamored by their own musings, leading to narcissistic gratification. Maroda (2002), arguing strongly for the inevitability of talking about the therapist's emotional re-actions once they are felt, wrote that intuition may be useful for experienced therapists but hardly for beginners.

The question has been raised whether relational therapy is an expression of New York-ish talkativeness (Bollas, 2015). Does the spontaneous dialogue impede the patient's need for reflection, dreaming, and fantasizing? Do re-lational therapists work in the secondary process, at the level of conscious interaction rather than staying in the unconscious (Bernstein, 1999)?

Consider the patient who recounts the latest insolences and indignities his partner has expressed. Should the therapist remain silent, waiting for a broader picture? Or side with the patient and express support? Validate his reactions? With full respect for all variation, a potential therapist response might be to line up with the patient. Not primarily to confirm but to react as expected to the stimulus value of the patient's narrative. However, the therapist approach would be made with full attention to the succeeding interaction, to upcoming doubts and hesitance. In the words of Maroda: "for the analyst to attempt to stifle her naturally occurring emotional re-sponses is to deprive the patient of exactly what he is desperately seeking, both to validate his own emotional responses and to encourage the feeling and naming of buried affects" (2002, p. 107).

It is apparent that self-disclosures may express the therapist's neediness for attention and not be helpful to the patient. The patient may express gratitude about the therapist's openness and hide, or perhaps not be aware of, subtle feelings that the therapist is invasive (Ghent, 1990; Slochower, 2017). Expressivity and restraint both have their time (Cooper, 2008).

In all interactions, however intimate they are, persons do not disclose all their feelings and fantasies. The question about judiciousness and skilfulness when self-disclosing is a matter of sensibility and common sense. A mother may be quite open, vulnerable, and tentative in discussing her feelings with a teenage child, but she would not disclose her intimate feelings about her husband in this conversation. We know the limits, or we try to. Psychotherapy is not a law trial, it is an attempt to use significant im-pressions and fantasies in order to further the patient's development (Aron, 1996; Beebe, Jaffe, & Lachmann, 1992).

David

A few days ago, David had been at his workplace. He took a cup of coffee and listened to the others. His workmates talked about a lecture they had been to recently. They had not asked him to participate, and David got the impression that they did not count on him anymore. They did not even apologize for not inviting him. He became extremely upset and went away without saying goodbye.

– So you felt really abandoned.
– They don't bother about me at all, they ignore me.
– Couldn't you have asked them about it?
– Are you stupid? You think I should ask them? They should ask me. You don't understand how insolent they are. You think I should ask them?
– Your anger spills over on me, it seems.
– Sometimes, I think you're just so analytic. You don't realize I was angry?
  Anne tries to capture what she feels. She really tries to empathize with David, but now she feels hurt. Her questions about what happened at the garage seem quite reasonable to her. Half spontaneously, half deliberately, Anne challenges David.
– I hear that you're angry at me also. And I understand that you felt abandoned by your work mates. But I do think that you overreacted. You've been on sick leave for several months and I think this was the first time you visited your workplace. Why should they invite you to the lecture?
– So you want me to feel ashamed for behaving impolitely.
  Anne decides to remain in her confrontative mode.
– That's not at all what I say. But I do think you react like the princess on the pea.

The dialogue develops into a somewhat heated discussion about David's reaction and Anne's perceived lack of understanding. After some bickering about different perspectives, Anne gets an uncanny feeling that she has a superiority that she is not comfortable with. She discloses her feelings about that. She suggests a role play where they change roles. David skilfully expresses Anne's view, and after that, they can talk about the way he feels not only abandoned but despised by his work mates. Together, they could work with David's feelings of sadness and hopelessness.

Anne's spontaneity is genuine. It may be due to her own personal issues. She may be too certain about the appropriateness of her reactions. Real conversations are influenced by various and not always transparent motives. Spontaneous talk relies on the immediate intuition. It is like downhill skiing. It is passion, it is not reflection. Reflection, afterthought, comes afterwards.

How to do in practice

If I want to understand how a person is experienced in relationships with other people, I can listen to how he describes his relationships with others. I may even get the opportunity to observe how he interacts with others. This is what therapists often do when they want to understand what relational difficulties a patient may have. A more immediate way is the therapist's own experience of being in relationship with the patient.

We can use the metaphor of understanding how a person plays tennis. It is possible to talk with him about how he plays, hear what strengths and weaknesses he thinks he has. Or to look at him playing with someone, observe how he meets the ball, how he seems to plan his game, and how hard his punches seem to be.

But the best way to understand his way of playing is by playing with him. When I try to handle his screwed-up serves and short balls, I know how it feels. And if I decide to play, I have to play for real. He may become angry at me, or disappointed. Or I at him. To really understand his playing style, I must try to take his serves and hit them back. If I just see them pass, it will not be a game.

Similarly, I need to be in real dialogue with the patient if I want to understand how he creates a relationship. I must become an engaged partner in the conversation. Sometimes playing tennis makes you angry at your opponent. Or impressed. Feelings are part of the play.

If the shared understanding of the patient's situation is furthered by modifications of the conventional rules and boundaries for talking therapies, there are no obstacles to develop mutual exploration except decency and a sense about what kind of relationship we have.

An illustration:

The patient has the impression that the therapist has hinted that he should separate. She does not think she has, although she thinks he should. But she also realizes that the patient is not easy to live with and she understands that he is afraid that he will not find anyone else to live with. She doesn't know if she should say anything about her thoughts, but when the patient starts talking about how scared he is of being alone, she says that maybe she would find it difficult to live with him because of his sometimes exaggerated self-esteem. She immediately regrets saying it when she realizes that the patient seems to be hurt. Perhaps she should try to say that she thinks he became hurt? The patient continues to look sad. She asks what he thinks, and he starts talking about always feeling alone and outside of the social context. She could have said many other things. What she said may seem clumsy in the rear-view window. But the fact that she said something and did not remain silent meant that they have a situation where they can work on problematic and constructive ways of relating.

Listening

Attentive listening is a fundamental approach in psychotherapy. Sometimes, however, therapeutic listening becomes formalized passivity. Silence may be not only an expression of respect for what the patient needs to say and a quiet curiosity about one's own reactions, but also an avoidance of things that ought to be said. Good therapy balances on the verge between attentive presence and appropriate challenge.

This is a balance. Although therapy conversation may sometimes sound like social talk (Hoffman, 2009b), there are times when "watching and waiting, maintaining a thoughtful inwardness" (Seligman, 2018, p. 132) may be required. Silence, reflection, and contemplation may also be called for. Bass (2014) argued for the therapist's right to remain silent ("a plea for a measure of private, quiet contemplation and spacious unhurried reverie", p. 664).

Structure and spontaneity

Although psychotherapy is based on formal and informal rules, no therapeutic interaction follows a script, not even when the therapist uses guidelines. It is at least to some extent improvised. If the therapist tries to figure out in advance how she should respond, she will not be accurately responsive (Watson & Wiseman, 2021).

In relational therapy, hope in the evolving process begets the structure. At a certain point, the therapist may find that she feels like joking with a one patient, whilst with another she may sense that it is important to appear formal and serious in order to gain confidence. Such clues, such action tendencies will direct the therapist's talk flow. She may try to formulate her feeling. Or her doubtfulness about being expressive.

Let us think that the therapist has the ambition to help the patient formulate himself. Listening and commenting seems ok to her, but not advising. A situation arises when the patient starts talking about changing jobs and the therapist thinks it would not be good at all if he did. He is constantly fleeing from the difficulties at his jobs. Should she say that? Or should she follow the patient's thoughts and feelings? Maybe she should help him clarify his feelings to his work mates, so he catches the reason why he wants to change. He is never able to stand up and get angry. It would be better for him to understand the situation than to change jobs. Could she say that? At what time? With how much emphasis?

These choices are there all the time. It is usually helpful not to think too long before speaking and at the same time try to be as wise as you can. The important thing is that if we are to work with the emotions in the relationship then we must not be fearful of them. We must dare to let them show up, pronounced. We must start from the idea that we are as smart as we are capable of being, say what seems reasonable and keep other feelings and thoughts to ourselves. It is in this spontaneous conversation that sometimes things that we had not thought may happen, that we surprise ourselves and our patient. Sometimes it gets really good, sometimes it gets crazy, sometimes we just pass over it.

By tradition, psychodynamic therapists leave room to the patient when the session starts. In longer therapies, the therapist may be open for roaming between different themes, hoping that the basic conflicts will emerge. In time-limited treatments, the therapist tries to understand the patient's material as expression of the agreed-upon conflict and turn the conversation in that direction.

In line with the flexible structure of relational therapy, there is no reason for the therapist not to take the initiative. In a situation where the patient does not come up with emotionally charged material, the therapist may comment on that. But she may also choose to connect to material from the last session. "When we met last week, you talked about your conflict with your boss. You seemed to be satisfied with how it ended but I continued reflecting about what you really felt". The rational may be to show that the patient remains in the therapist's mind, that the therapist has another perspective, that therapy is mutual work.

The creative process and framing

The therapist may be an expert on spontaneous, engaged talk, feeling reasonably confident that the therapeutic process has the potential to create its own structure, hoping that meaningful patterns will emerge. The patient, however, is not an expert of therapy processes. He may find open-ended talk confusing, without direction, even meaningless. He may hope the therapist will find a red thread in his complaints, understand the problem, and find a way forward. Especially in short contacts, a purely explorative stance of waiting for the patient's narratives to engender understandable problems may be felt to be frustrating by the patient.

In such situations, it may be important to frame the dialogue without removing its vitality. The most concrete way is to write a frame on the whiteboard and suggest with boxes and arrows to the patient what may be happening between them. Framing can also be made with words.

"You seem to feel that we move in different directions at every session. I have also that impression. However, I think that premature closure on what your problems are really about might impede our understanding. But I think that we should both feel confident that the process is moving in a constructive direction, and continuously evaluate if it is".

The therapist thus comments on the mutual work, reassuring that she and the patient are on the same page.

Framing meta-communication

Sometimes, it may be important to frame the spontaneity. An illustration from everyday life:

> The wife is depressed, sometimes she has suicidal thoughts. Her husband has tried to talk with her, encourage her, listen to her, argue with her. "Think about our child!", "I love you", "It will pass, sometimes you feel better", "There is no one as important as you for our child". After a while, he gets impatient, tired, fed up. He thinks it would be better if his wife moved to her mother so that he could take care of their child alone. Although she has not threatened explicitly, he is afraid she might do something with herself and their child while he is at work.
>
> He is afraid that he if comes with his suggestion directly, she will feel it as an attack on her motherhood. She is of no use to her child; she might just as well kill herself.
>
> He may say: "I want to share my thoughts with you. I realize you may feel upset, but I'll try to start with my own feelings and thoughts. ... What I'm saying now is not the only thoughts I have, but they are those that are hardest to formulate". He frames his statements. He announces that they belong to a specific mental space.

What does the therapist say in a similar situation? The patient constantly says that he does not want to live anymore; it would be better for everyone if he were dead. As soon as something comes up, he starts talking about suicidal thoughts. The therapist has tried to assess the risk of the patient's threats, she has tried to get the patient to agree on a suicide contract, she has tried to assess the risk if she talked about her frustration over the patient's constant threat. She feels trapped by the patient's threats; the patient does not find a way to reflect on her fear of suicide. They are in a mutual enactment.

How does this therapist talk about her feelings about what is going on between her and the patient? Sometimes the framing must be very clear. An attempt:

– I would like us to talk for a moment about how it is when the question of your suicidal thoughts comes up in our conversation. You've probably noticed that I get worried and a little cautious when we talk about them. Now I think it has become important that I talk about how things are between us. I get very frustrated when you take the suicide argument as soon as I suggest you could take more responsibility. It sometimes feels like you become threatening when I try to talk about you being able to talk with your husband seriously. It feels like you're running away from talking about suicide.

I hope you understand that I'm saying this because I have respect and trust in you. I feel quite nervous when I say it and of course I am afraid that you should say something about suicide. But it would feel dishonest not to tell you how annoyed I am.

One way to clarify that I as a therapist now want to talk about our relationship is to use an image. "Now I would like to stop for a while and think about what we would think if we had recorded our conversation and looked at it together. How do you think the last few minutes between us have been?" or "To get the right perspective on what we are doing, I would like us, metaphorically, to stand next to each other and look at us, perhaps as if from a height we look down on a landscape. To me it looks like a peacefulness that may not be so peaceful. What does it look like for you?"

The influence of the therapist and on the therapist

A reasonable reason for the therapist not to be talkative is that she may want to help the patient find his own ways and solutions. If the therapist discloses her opinions, experiences, or knowledge, she may feel that she obstructs the patient's possibility to develop agency in options and reflections.

Undoubtedly, there is a risk that a therapist may give limiting and uncalled-for views. However, a better point of departure is probably that the therapist does what a sensible and responsive person does. She gives advice and commentaries when fit. If she is wrong, she or the patient will discover it, sooner or later. Then, they have relational work ahead.

The unavoidable identification

Some professions are to a larger extent associated with aspects of the personal identity than others. A priest is a priest all the time, she cannot confess her belief in God in working hours and disclose that she is an atheist in her spare time. Actors and novelists use their private repertoire of emotions and life experiences when they perform or create works of art. In contrast, the plumber, the salesclerk, or the engine driver probably can leave the job when they have leisure time.

To what degree the profession is part of the personal identity has significance for comments about our work. If the plumber gets criticized for her way of putting together pipes, she can get angry that her professional skills are being questioned. But if the drain does not work, it is obvious that something is wrong. The plumber can do it right next time. If the novelist is criticized for his book, it will be much closer to his person. It is an aspect of his creativity, his way of perceiving life, that has been criticized. If the novel characters seem superficial, or the interaction between them lacks credibility, the author can feel that his person has been criticized. The plumber may have guilt feelings about badly performed jobs; the novelist probably becomes ashamed when the novel is seen as uninteresting.

Therapists' immediacy self-disclosures are closer to their ongoing self-experience than narratives from their life. Many therapists could keep at a distance a patient's comments if she has disclosed how she handled a difficult situation with a teenager; questioning the confusion she discloses as a reaction to the patient's ongoing talk may be more difficult to take. Immediacy reactions are not neutral reports about the therapists' thoughts and life. They move on the border between what seems possible to say and what should perhaps not be said.

Ethical issues

The private side of therapy comes to the fore when we realize that meaningful therapy always touches ethical dilemmas (Drozek, 2015). An illustration:

- I won't leave my flat in the evenings. There are all kinds of strange young men around.
  The therapist has been active in an organization for refugees and is eager to help persons get a more positive picture of immigrants.
- It might be good for you to not to give in to your fears. I think you may exaggerate the dangers.
- My friend was almost raped some weeks ago. Easy for you who is an older man. Women nowadays are always in danger.
  The therapist knows a number of young foreign men and has been active in helping them to find native friends.
- You seem to have a lot of fantasies about them.
- That's not fantasies. All my friends are scared. I think some of you well-meaning established persons think that we should take all the trouble with rapists, and you continue talking nicely with them. It's upsetting.
- You think I don't really care about you, that I just see your problems as a phobia.
- I do.

The conversation continues with mutual considerations about the situation for young women in places with many young men from other countries. They successively find out the differences in their opinions. However, the patient leaves the session with a feeling that the therapist never will understand what it in reality means to be scared about being raped. The therapist knows that he will not be able to know in depth what his patient feels.

Personal and private

A distinction is often made between private and personal regarding what is possible for the therapist to say about herself to the patient. Personal usually means information that is public or easily attainable, private could be that the therapist considers separating from her partner.

But reflect on this dialogue:

- I don't think we sleep with each other more than once a month.
- It sounds like quite seldom.

- I don't like it anymore. I don't think it's a problem.
- It may be different, but to me it sounds like rare and something we should reflect on.

Where does the therapist get this knowledge from? From statistics on how often people sleep with each other? Perhaps more likely from her own experience. When therapists decide what should be addressed as problems or as questions to reflect on, they use the experience available to them, often their own (Hoffman, 1983; Maroda, 2002).

The situation is somewhat similar to the actor's. When she gets the manuscript, the words are on the paper. The actor has to make herself available for the text. She offers her life experiences, her personality to get the energy and the dynamics that make the performance possible. If the actor just reads the manuscript aloud, it will not become credible. But if she lets her person take over the role, it will not be theatre. The challenge is to enrich the role with one's own life without letting the life take over the role.

The task for the therapist is similar. She has a role to play. The role is constantly changing in accordance with the patient's developing expectations and fears. The therapist makes herself available for the role. She offers her experience, her life, and her emotions to make the interaction possible. Making herself available means opening doors to her interior. But which door should be opened, what should be shown? We cannot know, we can only know that some doors must open for the therapy to become vital.

An artwork may express the artist's fears and hopes, her inner life. The concrete expression is one of many possibilities. When relational situations emerge between patient and therapist, they are not copies of previous experiences. They are new expressions, with a tension between the found and the created. In this intersubjective potential space, where meanings are created and transformed, self-disclosures have their place. They are earnest attempts to formulate a concrete experience between therapist and patient; but they are attempts, open to interpretations like a work of art. They are invitations to find new meanings in the interaction.

In solution-focused therapies, the question of privacy limits is often uncontroversial. If the patient wants to send a postcard from his holiday resort, it does not influence the common work of learning how to regulate impulsiveness or expose to anxiety-provoking situations. But the more the therapeutic relationship moves in the direction of a potential intersubjective space, the more important will the boundaries towards the "mundane" world become. The real emotional engagement, and the play in the potential space, emphasizes the personal importance of the relationship.

Let us think that the patient asks whether it would be all right to send a text message every day about his emotional condition. The therapist knows that the patient is lonely and has often considered whether to offer more contact, sometimes with a pang of bad conscience. She accepts the patient's question about text messages but says she will not respond. After a few days, the messages reek of loneliness feelings. The therapist regrets that she did not refuse the question. She realizes that the patient may be provocative, but she also thinks that he is indeed very lonely. All kinds of fantasies come up in her.

Was it a mistake to accept the patient's question? It would be easy to decide on a general rule, like "never", or "under specific circumstances". In relational therapy, the answer is in the process, in the material that is created. The therapist's thought: "How could I be so stupid?" is part of the therapy, potentially disclosable. The process implies that therapeutic dialogues sometimes go awry, the participants become uncertain whether they are on a constructive track or not. They may balance spontaneity with reflection, thoughtfulness with boldness. It is like cycling, you cannot keep the balance if the bike does not move forward. Similarly, the conversation loses its suspense unless what is said is challenged by a new, not always finished, thought.

15 Be mindful of the affective interplay

The tool

It is in our affective relations with other people that we both understand who we are and get our psychological problems. Affects are the driving force of psychological suffering and wellbeing; they carry the potential for therapeutic change. Emotional communication is the way humans understand themselves and manage their relationships (Tronick, 1989).

The therapist's main challenge is to become aware of and to use the emotions in the therapeutic interaction in a helpful way. The emotional atmosphere in the relationship is sometimes obvious, but it may also be hardly perceptible, subtle, with elusive nuances. There is usually an interactional aspect of emotion recognition: my feelings give indications of what you may feel. When the child is confused about what he feels, there is hopefully a parent who not only tries to help the child formulate what he feels but who can use her own emotional compass to find directions. Emotions may seem private but in human development they get their shape and meaning in the emotional interaction with others.

The relational tool is openness and curiosity about feelings that arise, in the therapist and in the patient. It is important to strike a balance between establishing a trustful and collaborative atmosphere and simultaneously tolerate and stimulate curiosity about less wished-for feelings. No emotions are better than others, all emotions are meaningful. If there is no feeling, the challenge is to find one. If there is a feeling, pay attention to it! The therapist should help her patient catch, clarify, nuance, and give words to his emotions and to articulate her own feelings about what is going on in the relationship, with caution and sensitivity. And with a genuine willingness to share. The guiding principle is to follow the feeling rather than the narrative, thought, or activity.

The purpose

Emotions make life understandable and vital. They inform us about the meaning of what we experience, they give life to relationships. When we

DOI: 10.4324/9781003026914-15

cannot experience emotions or express them, when we are only open to a few emotions and a narrow range of intensity, we have problems in living. The purpose of this tool is to increase the patient's emotional awareness, his ability to recognize emotions, to express them, to reflect on them, and to be vitalized by them. As interventions that focus on the patient's interpersonal problems outside therapy may stimulate intellectual rather than emotional work (Gabbard & Westen, 2003), the actual interaction is a golden place for work with affects.

The dilemma

Affects are infectious. The feeling evoked in the recipient is not, however, always the feeling in the sender. Anger in the sender may engender fear or shame in the recipient. It may be hard to disentangle what the sender really feels. Although the therapist may have hunches about the patient's reactions or ask for them, the immediate "data" is her own emotions.

Feelings are more persuasive than thoughts; often we get stuck in them. Once you become engaged by a feeling, you tend to keep to it even if, at second thought, other feelings may be more evident. Consider the situation when you become overwhelmed by an intensive feeling, let it be anger, envy, or sadness. When someone else tries to figure out what you "really" feel, it is often difficult to let go of the original feeling. "Leave my feelings to myself". You may want to stay in them, even enjoy them.

Feelings are not worth much if they do not engage, but it is hard to know when they have got stuck. This is true also for the therapist. Are my feelings, or the shared feelings, really helpful to the patient or are they idiosyncratic in a negative way to me or us?

There is a fine balance between the ditch of becoming too engaged, perhaps taking over and controlling the emotional formulations, and the ditch of becoming too passive and not responding to the patient's feelings in a living way.

Principles

Affects are central to human interaction. And not only in engaged interaction; in everyday encounters, we constantly, although often out of awareness, handle the nature and degree of emotions between us. If the feeling does not come by itself, we may help it emerge. If I talk with someone on the bus, I wait for the feeling to appear in order to become engaged. What is comforting, interesting, upsetting? We gradually find out what kind of relation we have with the other by listening for the feeling between us. Do I feel happy with her, embarrassed, do I regret that I started the conversation? Emotions are the carrier of meaningfulness in our relationships. Ability to differentiate among emotions, to perceive their granularity, is associated with greater resilience against mental problems (Kashdan, Barrett & McKnight, 2015).

Affects are the driving force of therapeutic change (Aafjes-van Doorn & Barber, 2017; Dahl et al., 2014; Dahl, Ulberg, Friis, Perry, & Høglend, 2016; Foa et al., 2019; Greenberg & Pascual-Leone, 2006; Jaycox et al., 1998). Therapeutic schools emphasize various aspects but the ability to be aware of affects and to tolerate them is seen as essential in most of them. In exposure treatment, the technique consists of habituating the patient to fear of external stimuli or to increase his tolerance for uncomfortable feelings in the context of a safe relationship with a therapist. In humanistic therapies, the therapist's task is to help the patient become curious about disavowed feelings and to help him explore new ones. In mindfulness meditation, a main aim is to tolerate feelings without pushing them away or evaluating them.

Emotion regulation

In the therapy world, there is a tension between models that advocate regulating feelings and those that emphasize becoming aware of them and tolerating their intensity. In the Unified Protocol treatment, the aim is to tolerate and regulate (Barlow & Farchione, 2017). In MBT, lukewarm emotional intensity makes mentalizing optimal (Gunderson, Bateman, & Kernberg, 2007), in DBT emotion regulation tools are taught to the patient (Linehan, 2015). For some patient groups, like persons with autism, a low arousal approach is recommended (McDonnell et al., 2015). In dynamic therapies, affect experiencing is usually proposed; the patient's access to strong emotions is key to change (Davanloo, 1995; Fosha, 2000).

A problem with this discussion is that it often does not take non-verbal mutual regulation into account (Ramseyer, 2020). Interaction, in psychotherapy and elsewhere, takes place in the symbolic and the subsymbolic systems (Bucci, 2018; Schore & Schore, 2008). Rather than trying to regulate the subsymbolic, affective system, the therapist may attend to and reflect on it.

An illustration:
The patient is a 30-year-old man who repeatedly has strong outbursts of feelings. His partner as well as his friends tell him that it is basically ok with strong emotions but in the end, it becomes too much. His therapist has validated his need for emotional expression. At the last session, the patient was extremely angry at the therapist because the session before had been cancelled with short notice. The therapist apologized and tried to get him reflect on the intensity of his anger. The patient became even angrier and rushed out through the door. The therapist waited and after some minutes the patient returned. He was still very angry and threatened to end the therapy, accusing the therapist of not bothering about his schedule. Similar things had happened previously. The patient looks at the therapist:

- You look angry. What kind of therapy is this? Am I not allowed to show that I feel frustrated?
  The therapist felt serious but not angry.
- I wouldn't say that I'm angry. But I think we must understand what happens.
- To me it's unproblematic. I had moved an important appointment and then you cancel. Of course I get angry.

Who's feelings?

A leading idea in psychoanalytic therapy since the 1950s has been that aspects of the patient's inner world can be understood by the therapist's countertransference reactions. Winnicott (1949) argued for an *objective countertransference* meaning that any therapist would react in the same way to a particular behaviour; *projective identification* means that disavowed feelings in the patient without conscious awareness become projected into the therapist and experienced by her (Ogden, 1989).

Relational theory takes another perspective. The question "Does the irritation come from the patient or is it mine?" is not a relational question (Govrin, 2016). The irritation is in me, so it is mine. But it has emerged in our relationship; it is specific to the relationship. I may have my reasons to become irritated, the patient may have his reasons to provoke me. But the feelings emerge in our relationship. "Conceptually, it is a process of collision and negotiation between the patient's and analyst's self-states that slowly fosters recognition of each other's (and one's own) dissociated aspects of self … a negotiated, nonlinear dialectic of dissonance and restructuring that is at once so clinically foundational and so unpredictably messy" (Bromberg, 2012a, p. 9).

Affects emerge in relationships. Although I may walk alone with my despair, I have others in my mind. Affects are used for communication. May I comfort you? Do you notice that I look worried? Are you scared that I think you are stupid? "Emotions are not inner states that we experience only individually or that we have to decode in others, but instead are primarily shared states that we experience through interbodily affectivity, often without verbal articulation" (BCPSG, 2018b, p. 302).

Facilitative therapist feelings

The relational stance is engaged curiosity. As noted in Chapter 4, this stance differs from the idea of a normative facilitative approach in, for instance, person-centred therapy. The humanistic idea of a therapist who is empathic, emotionally present, and non-possessively warm is of course a general basis for all therapies. But more prioritized is curiosity about potential lack of empathy and warmth.

Distinctions between different emotional therapist approaches may be subtle. Is it possible, for instance, to be both authentic, and to show unconditional positive regard, two keywords in the humanistic stance, at the same time (Wachtel, 2008)? It is instructive to compare the relational approach with Fosha's description of AEDP, a short-term dynamic therapy. "We explore the client's receptive affective experience – or lack thereof – of the therapist's care, empathy or validation" (Fosha, Thoma & Yeung, 2019, p. 7). In this perspective, the therapist offers a (normative) approach of care and empathy and explores together with the patient his way of using it. The difference with relational therapy may seem subtle. In relational therapy, therapist empathy is not presupposed, it is a relational possibility. Lack of empathy is a also a potential intersubjective experience in therapy. The stance is curiosity on the patient's complex reaction to the therapist's complex feelings.

The therapist's role in evoking feelings

Sometimes, the therapy dialogue seems to lack feelings. The patient is devoid of them, the therapist finds it hard to access them. The conversation is felt as sterile and barren. The therapist may attempt to help the patient describe and detail situations when she thinks emotions could have been evoked, to no avail. She may try to detect her own feelings, without result. By challenging for detailed descriptions, the dialogue may develop. An illustration:

The parents of the patient were extremely occupied with their career jobs during his adolescence. In the summers, they used to leave their house for weeks, letting the patient take care for it.

– Didn't you feel lonely when they were away?
– I didn't bother much. They called me sometimes.
– You were quite young. And the summer when your sister had all those parties in your house, and you had to tidy up after them?
– It sounds tough but I didn't think much about it.
  The therapist has never been in such a situation herself, but she can imagine the lonely boy in the big house and the sister sometimes coming home.
– There's something in your story that really catches me. It seems to me that you're not very moved by your memories. But for some reason I am. It's like I see the house, big and empty, and you strolling around without purpose and activating yourself just to have something to do. Am I wrong?
– I think you're right. I think it was pretty lonely some days.
  The therapist gets some confirmation, but she feels that her sense of loneliness is much bigger than that of her patient's.
– I would have felt left and, well, perhaps angry.
– That's not the kind of person I was. I didn't think much. You're a therapist, I guess you have more feelings.
– Could be true.

- You're trying to palm off your feelings on me. I'm not the kind of person you are.
- I guess anyone would feel somewhat left in that situation.
- I don't think I did. I think you're imposing your ideas on me. I didn't feel that lonely.

  At this moment, the focus has changed from the patient's memories to the interaction. The therapist has to consider whether her view of the situation is in some way idiosyncratic to her or if it feels justified and adequate.
- So, you think I impose my ideas on you?
- Yes, you do. I feel pressed about it.
- Could you say more?
- Sometimes, I think you just want to squeeze me like a lemon.
- That sounds unpleasant.
- I don't understand how you can know what I ought to feel.

The dialogue has moved to another place. Now, the patient has feelings, but towards the therapist rather than about his summer situation. We might of course wonder whether they could reflect repressed feelings towards the parents, but a better option is to stay in the ongoing relationship between therapist and patient. The therapist does not provoke feelings, she engages in the discussion with the patient and is open to what may come.

Working with trauma

No life is lived without psychological traumas (Kohut, 1971). They are a part of life. At times, the emotional load exceeds our capacity to manage and respond in adequate and constructive ways. Some persons experience more severe, more painful hardships, or more continuous abuse than others. Some traumas are disastrous and make indelible impressions like war experiences and rapes, or cumulative adverse experiences during are long time. Traumas with a human perpetrator have more deleterious effects and lead to PTSD diagnoses to a larger extent than non-interpersonal traumas (Briere, Agee & Dietrich, 2016). The variation in trauma experiences and their sequelae is large. All traumas evoke complicated feelings, trauma consequences often imply that emotions as warded off or get overwhelming, trauma therapy is emotionally trying for both patient and therapist.

- Karen had been assaulted one day when she went home from school by a man who forced her to oral sex. She was eight years old. Her mother called the police, Karen was interrogated, but the police never found the man. Her mother had felt desperate. Karen's memory later was that her mother was more concerned with her own feelings than with Karen's experience. Karen soon stopped thinking about the incident. In adolescence, she had dreams about repulsive sexual situations and, at occasions, anxiety attacks. On a visit to a school psychologist, she realized that the situation in childhood might have significance for her symptoms. After a treatment focused on the incident, her symptoms disappeared. Later in life, when she had marital problems, her therapist helped her reflect on her relationship with her mother, and particularly what happened between them when she was raped.

The therapist strongly felt that the mother had not been empathic enough with her daughter. However, by and by, it struck her that Karen had a very large, perhaps too large, need to talk about the rape. At first, she had guilt feelings as she realized that Karen had really been badly abused. When she finally approached the subject, it became meaningful for Karen to talk about how people whom she trusted were not as attentive to her problems as she hoped. She was quite disappointed with her husband in this regard and found it possible to talk with him when the therapist's disclosure of her feelings had been worked through.

- Throughout her childhood, Anne has seen her father drunk from time to time. Sometimes he threatened to hit someone in the family. Anne was the one in the family who could talk with him when he was drunk. She found ways to keep him reasonably calm. She felt proud of that and was often not aware of the fear and anger that she also felt. As an adult, she had some difficult experiences in relationships. Her relational style seemed to be to provoke her partners until they got exasperated and, on some occasions, hit her. Intermittently, she also abused alcohol.

  At the start of the therapy, the therapist felt sorry for her. After an incident when Anne became angry at the therapist and the therapist slowly realized that her own mild reaction was in fact rather odd, she got really irritated and told Anne with clarity that she felt hurt. There followed a series of conflicts between them. The enactments with a still sometimes overly kind therapist were finally worked through. Anne left therapy with better ability to avoid acting in aggressive situations and a healthy assertiveness.

- Sven's parents enjoyed living close to nature and wanted their children to be part of this lifestyle. He and his siblings were not allowed to have mobile phones or computers; his parents wanted them to play with things they found in the forest. The family wore home-knitted sweaters and caps. Sven was teased by his classmates for clothes they thought were funny. Children who had been at Sven's home talked about how odd it was there. During his school time, Sven was ambivalent about the family's lifestyle. Sometimes he was proud, but often he wished for a more normal life. After secondary school, he opted for a progressive art school. He was unsuccessful in his creative work and had to leave the school. After trying several menial jobs without finding them stimulating enough, he decided to apply to a teacher college. He also started therapy in order to understand why his relationships always ended after a few weeks.

In his therapy, he became occupied by the therapist's private life and tried to figure out her political and religious values. He found out that she was much engaged in a political movement that had taken a stand against abortion. Sven tried to get hold of all information he could about this group. He tried to use the sessions to talk about politics. To begin with, the therapist was irritated by Sven's snoopiness and lack of interest in his complicated background. However, when the therapist decided to discuss moral issues with Sven, she felt strongly that their dialogue became interesting and fruitful. Sven could get in touch with his bewilderment and anger at his childhood life.

The witness

With trauma patients, the therapist often gets the position of witness. To hear about traumas is to be offered the possibility to engage in the patient's experiences. Empirical studies show the importance of the therapist for the patient's trust (Sandberg, Gustafsson, & Holmqvist, 2017).

An illustration shows the complexity of the therapist's situation:

The patient had been exposed to severely traumatic experiences during the civil war in his home country. He had been raped repeatedly and he had also been subjected to mock executions. He was plagued with permanent tiredness, nightmares, and invasive images. The therapist asked him to relate in detail would he had been exposed to. The patient describes how several men had penetrated him anally with a broom stick. The patient is clearly very affected by his description, crying silently at times. He sits with closed eyes. When he opens them, he looks attentively at the therapist.

–   You look frightened.
    The therapist feels exposed by the patient, embarrassed. She is uncertain about what to say.
–   I am very much touched by what you're talking about. I continue to listen.
    The patient sits quiet for a while.
–   I wonder how it feels to listen. Sometimes I think people try to keep a façade. They listen but they can't understand.
    The therapist decides to follow the patient.
–   It's true, I guess. I try to understand, and I do get shocked. But I haven't been there.
–   I wonder if I have. Physically I was there. I cried and I was afraid. I thought I'd die. But I don't know, in some way I kept it away.
–   And what happens now?
–   I became occupied with what I saw in your eyes. I thought I saw sympathy.
–   That's what I felt.
    The therapist gets tears in her eyes, she tries to hold them back
–   You were so vulnerable then, and you still are.

The dialogue moves to a place where the feelings between patient and therapist are in focus. They continue to explore the patient's shame over having been a victim and not having overcome it.

Traumatic experiences mean that the victim's trust in people has been damaged. The perpetrator has destroyed the belief in people's good will and intentions. In the presence of the therapist, the patient may dare to face his memories. The therapist's affective sensitivity for the attachment situation and the patient's tolerance for painful feelings decides the result (Russell, 1998). It cannot, however, be predicted how the therapist will react. Engagement may mean very different things.

Secondary traumatization

Therapists tend to answer in the affirmative when asked whether they can stand listening to patient stories about sexual and other abuse. This is in a way surprising. To listen to stories about how a perpetrator attacks a defenseless victim without compassion or respect should not be easy. However, professional role expectations require the therapist to stand on the patient's side and endure his feelings with him.

Many therapists who work with trauma victims develop secondary traumatization. The closer to the abused person's experience and the more concrete the story is, the stronger the listener's reaction will be, and the more difficult it will be to remain untouched. Becoming emotionally engaged by abuse and other traumas that patients have experienced makes the trust of fellow humans to falter or burst also for therapists. They may experience recurring nightmares, intrusive thoughts or images, depression, and fatigue. On the outside, the therapist may appear competent and well-functioning, but upon closer acquaintance, anxiety and depressive feelings rage.

Trauma work and the potential space

Traumas make things with persons. They colour the survivor's capacity to tolerate new hardships, potentially making him or her more vulnerable for anxiety and depression. Memories of them may hide in dissociated rooms, they may hijack the subject, making the victim a perpetrator. A common consequence of traumas is shattered attachment security, leading to problematic interpersonal behaviour.

Sometimes, patients report experiences that seem unbelievable. The traumas that the patient describe have an extreme character, the therapist may find it hard to be confirmative and empathic with the patient because she feels uncertain about the truthfulness; she may think that the patient fables. But she also realizes that she may become defensive because the horror is so terrible.

On such occasions, the potential space stance is useful. Engaged interest, but outside the question of truth. There is always a relational implication of what the patient tells, a wish to involve the therapist in something, although the significance may be unclear. The narrative is an invitation to enter the potential room. Or rather one of the rooms, one of the connections between a room in the patient and a room in the therapist.

Emotional agency in trauma patients

To be exposed for traumatic violence implies that the victim's subjective agency is threatened. It is important for the trauma patient to regain or develop his experience of subjectivity (Ogden, 1992; Stern, 1985). Emotional change comes successively. Already from birth child and the parent to find a rhythm in their emotional interaction (Fonagy, Gergely, Jurist & Target, 2005; Trevarthen, 1977). The child becomes acquainted with its own feeling patterns. For the traumatized patient, it may be a long way to come back to the ongoing agency feelings.

The patient has been abused by his wife, both mentally and physically. He is a kind person; he usually withdraws and excuses her. He comes from a family where his father used to beat up his mother and he had to console her. Lately, his wife has begun hitting him and humiliate him publicly. The therapist wonders why he does not become angry at her.

–   Can we talk about what happened in last week?
–   We had some friends for dinner. She got drunk and started insulting me. She said that I'm a lousy lover, that she's never loved me, that she can't stand me.
–   What did you feel?
–   I was ashamed of her. I think our guests thought that she made a fool of herself.
–   Did they say that?
–   No, they left quite early. Then she drank more and started boxing on me. She even clocked me one.
–   How was that for you?
–   I tried to calm her.
–   Did you get angry?
–   I don't really get angry. I try just to calm her. I don't want to be like she is. I think she is sick; she needs help.

The therapist attempts to help the patient access more anger. The patient makes his best but does not feel any real anger.

The therapist reflects on the situation. Although she tries to be friendly, she thinks that her insistence on anger feelings may be felt as a critique.

–   When I think of it, I realize that I may sound critical. As if I think you ought to feel anger.
–   Well, I guess you have good intentions.

- It sounds as if there was one more thought in that.
- Sometimes I wonder if you think I'm a coward.

There is some truth in what the patient says.

David

David wants to talk about his relationship with his mother when he was a child. Anne sometimes has the impression that David avoids dealing with his current problems by insisting on talking about his childhood. Although they initially agreed that it might be positive for David to reflect on childhood disappointments, Anne has become doubtful about how beneficial it is for him.

Now David wants to talk about his loneliness as a child. Sometimes he was with his uncle when his mother worked, but often he was at home alone. Sometimes he was scared when he was alone. He used to hear things from the stairs and then he imagined that someone came for a call and he did not know if he would dare to open the door. Anne could easily imagine his fear in the situation. David talked for a while and Anne asked questions to help him remember specific situations. However, it was not easy to get David become really concrete. The sounds in the stairs were as far as he came, otherwise it was mostly about how he had thought about what Mom was doing and when she would come home.

Anne understood that this must have been hard for him, but still she did not feel that she was getting into David's story. David had often talked about this. It was certainly important for him, but she had the impression that he had talked about this so often that the story had found its traces, the words had become solidified and without affect.

- It must have been difficult for you. I remember how I felt when I was afraid of what might happen when I was a child. But when I thought about my reaction to your narrative, it struck me that it is as if I'm not really getting into your story. It feels ready-made when you tell it. It is like a tale from your childhood, you don't seem to be very touched when you talk.
- It's not the first time I talk about this.
- I thought so. Although your story has a gripping content, I was not really caught.

Silence for some seconds

- I feel lonely when you say that. My memories are not easy, and I don't know how to get you understand how tough it was. I don't kVnow how to tell you about it.
  Anne thinks about whether to express compassion with David's loneliness or to point to the lack of feeling once more.

- It's as if you were behind a screen or a glass, as if I know you are there but do not see the contours so I could know who you are.
- Yes, I'm kind of diffuse for everyone. My boss is decent, but he doesn't see me. And my wife, she has seen me but now she only sees a depressed man.
- And I only see a man who comes with the childhood stories that he usually tells. That really sounds lonely.
- It has always been like that. I have been there, but no one has seen me. *Now, the words feel a lot more genuine and believable to Anne. David's words are saturated with feeling. He is struggling to find words that fit what he feels.*
- No one has seen me, you say. I've talked with you for quite some time. Is it that you are disappointed in me for not understanding what it was like for you?
- I've probably turned it off. I don't expect people to understand. Perhaps I don't understand myself.
- And what do you feel about that?
- I'm on the outside.

Anne struggles to catch a feeling and finds it in their actual relationship rather than in David's history.

How to do in practice

Affective reactions are private. When you watch a movie, you often find that your feelings do not match your partner's, at least when you attempt to be nuanced about them. The interplay in therapy may evoke feelings that on the surface may seem general but, when scrutinized, are unique to the actual dyad.

These unique feelings are precious for the patient's development. Imagine that the patient tells you about how his wife has betrayed him. He has already talked with his friends. One of them is upset on behalf of the patient, another thinks it was time for the patient to get rid of her, and the third insists that he is more sad than he expresses.

When the therapist hears about it, she wonders why the patient seems so restrained. She feels confused as to what his feelings really are. She tells him about her impression. He looks even more tense. She thinks about the possibility to get under his surface by suggesting that he might be angry, or sad. But she also thinks it is important for him not to be rushed into formulating feelings. Some seconds elapse. The patient starts to talk about his feeling that people use his situation to ventilate their own ideas about separations. He has the feeling that people like sensations and they would love to use his current situation to share feelings with him. The fact is that he does not know what he feels. He feels numb, like when a part of the body has lost its sensitivity. After having formulated this feeling and his disappointment about being used, he slowly starts to find his feelings about his partner's behaviour. To find feelings is a subtle exploratory challenge.

The therapist's feelings

An important goal is to help the patient find the range of his feelings, the nuances. One way for the therapist is to explore and disclose her own feelings. Does this mean that the therapist has to be familiar with a spectrum of feelings, to be able to respond with emotional richness and clarity and not to avoid any feelings? Obviously not. All therapists have lacunae in their perception of emotions. They have their favourite and their feared feelings. They are as dependent on the ongoing emotional interaction as the patient. The patient does not need a therapist who has no blind spots. He needs a therapist who attempts to become aware of and to formulate her feelings, who is surprised by the patient's feelings and by her own.

However much the therapist tries to hide her feelings, the patient will attempt to get an idea of them; they will be visible in implicit and subtle ways (Maroda, 2002). Sometimes the therapist decides to describe feelings, often a good base for mutual reflection. A more stimulating move may be for the therapist to show her struggle to find out what she feels. The right words for feelings are seldom easy to find. Genuine emotional interaction emerges when the participants share their attempts to find them. An illustration:

In high school, the patient was abused sexually by a group of boys. She has cut herself since she was 17. Although being lesbian, she has prostituted herself to men during the last year. At the last session, she comes with a bandage around her forearm. A few evenings before, she sat in her bathtub with a razor blade and tried to cut herself in her arm with the intention to kill herself. When she realized that the wound that she cut along her arm would not cause her death, she went to the hospital's emergency room.

When she comes to the therapist, she has figured out how to cut herself in order to die the next time she tries.

– Do you want to see the wound?
  Before the therapist has time to respond, she rolls up her sleeve, takes the bandage away, and shows the wound.
– I tried to find the artery, so I had to dig around a bit. But I failed.
  The therapist feels disgusted. The wound is quite deep. But the therapist does not say anything about her reaction. The patient puts back the bandage. The therapist uses the remaining time to try to help the patient understand what feelings prompted her to this, without much success. During the next few days, the image of the wound comes to the mind of the therapist from time to time. At the next session, she decides to talk about it.
– I have thought quite a lot about what happened last time. You asked me if I wanted to see but then you showed me the wound before I had time

to respond. It made quite a strong impression on me; it has in fact popped up in my mind from time to time since then. So I wanted to tell you what I felt about it. … I'm not quite certain, really, it's kind of hard to find the words. The first thing, I think, is that I felt sorry for you. But then, I also felt disgusted and rather angry at you. You didn't give me a chance to respond. My feeling was that you forced your wound on me. What do you feel when I say this?

– I don't know.
– I realize that I may sound like a critical parent. Perhaps you think I ought to see it, that I shouldn't be critical but sympathetic. Or perhaps you wanted me to become angry. … It's odd, I realize that I become occupied by what you want from me. Simply, I did get scared.
– I saw that. I don't know why I showed you. I wanted you to know and to share, I guess.

The session continues with explorations about what feelings the description of the cutting event and the demonstration of the wound evoked in both of them.

Anxiety

Patients with anxiety symptoms constitute a considerable share of patients being treated in primary care and psychiatric clinics. Exposure is the standard treatment although there are examples of effective psychoanalytic therapies (Milrod et al., 2016; Svensson et al., 2021). Although people around persons with anxiety problems often react with frustration and anger, therapy is usually seen as the individual's own duty.

An illustration:
Martin had anxiety problems since his teens. He had grown up with his mother who had often criticized him verbally. He had also for some years been harassed in school. His mother knew it but insisted that he go to school even when he was scared. Now, in his late twenties, he lived with a girlfriend. He had often anxiety feelings, particularly in social situations. His therapist had attempted to help him in a number of ways. Primarily, she had encouraged him to expose himself to situations that evoked discomfort. The situations varied but they were often of a social nature. He had tried to go to the library and to shopping malls. He seldom succeeded; often he had to leave. His therapist insisted that he should stay, that he should not avoid the anxiety and discomfort. He tried but failed.

The therapist became frustrated. She started thinking that he did not take his assignments seriously. She hinted to him about her feeling. He became quite angry. Nobody understands how he tries. His girlfriend threatens to leave him. His mother never understood how serious the mobbing was. The rest of the therapy contact is spent on his feelings of abandonment and his understanding of others' reactions to him. The anxiety dissipates.

The right feeling

How does the therapist know that her feeling is helpful and constructive? Another therapist might have experienced other feelings. It is important to be aware that there are no correct feelings. The goal is to explore an array of feelings, to tolerate all kinds of them.

The patient, a man in the middle age, wanted to talk about his relationship to his wife. After some hesitation, he told his younger therapist that he did not sleep with his wife any longer. With a lot of discomfort, he admitted that although she was attractive, he did not get an erection. Her wife had tried to help him, but then he felt even more shameful and turned away from her. The therapist became embarrassed by the patient's apparent difficulty to talk about his unsuccessful attempts. She tried to be as direct as she mastered, but she did feel abashed. Both of them tried, none of them were courageous. After some time, she realized that she and her patient had created an emotional atmosphere that was not only characterized by shyness but also by warmth and tenderness. She talked with him about it. He agreed. Encouraged by this, she starts asking him about how his wife tries to seduce him. He becomes ostensibly provoked and responds vaguely. She insists but realizes that they are not on the same page. She comments on that. He says with some effort that he hates to have to talk about sexual feelings. His wife has made a number of attempts, and he just doesn't stand it.

The illustration shows how feelings that come up in the conversation evolve in their own tracks. The point is to follow them.

16 Attend to the common potential space

The tool

Interactions between persons take place in different relational modes. Potential space is a mode of possibilities. Although the character of the emotional atmosphere may be as hard to detect as the water for the fish, the therapist should try to use her relational palps to perceive potential playfulness, creativity, and curiosity or restrain and lack of freedom. The potential space is found but also created. The squiggle game is a metaphor for it; Winnicott initiated the play but let it evolve on its own premises. The therapist should have tolerance to let it grow at the same time as she contributes to its growth. If the intersubjective space is open enough, it may be a cradle for creative relating.

The purpose

Relationships may be described in different ways. They may be characterized by their balance of power and valence, by different degrees of energy and agency, affects and relational freedom. They may be creative, vitalizing, and open for reflection and fantasy (Aron, 2006; Ogden, 1985; Winnicott, 1971a), or rigid, foreseeable, narrow, and one-dimensional (Jacobs, 1991; Lyons-Ruth, 1999; McLaughlin, 1991). Potential space is one variant of experiencing the interaction. The purpose of tending the potential space is that it opens for the development of new ways of understanding history, new ways of finding relational possibilities, new ways of experiencing affect. It is the place where it is possible to play with reality (Fonagy & Target, 2007). "What if ... I would take a cup of tea at your kitchen table, ... think of you when we do not meet, ... be really disappointed with you". Thoughts can be played with.

The dilemma

The potential space is a space for play. Play is never intended to be constructive, forward-looking, solution oriented. Play is for the special kind of

DOI: 10.4324/9781003026914-16

earnestness that imbues art, fiction, and shared fantasizing. It is not meant to solve problems, not even to identify them. Perhaps to express dilemmas in life. No one would play with a prescribed dialogue or purpose. So – how do we know that the therapeutic work is constructive when we are in the potential space mood?

Principles

The potential space is one among several different ways of experiencing a relationship. The special importance of the potential space has to do with its potential as a place for creativity and change. The tie to culture that Winnicott made is felicitous as it shows its special character: a serious place for the imagination.

Play does not usually evolve on demand. Conditions can be arranged but the true feeling comes by itself. I can start reading a novel, but I cannot know if it will take hold of me. There are times when the play experience does not arise even though we are prepared for it. After watching a movie for 15 minutes, I may realize that I will not get into it. The potential space does not emerge.

There is an allurement in relational work that may be hard to avoid. The focus on the interplay, with the co-created possibilities, may become too fascinating. The risk is that the work becomes only fantasy, pretend mode, that the ties to reality are severed. How does the therapist know when potential space becomes pretend mode? The usual indications are fatigue, loss of interest, dullness. Attention to loss of creativity in the therapeutic work is, however, only one side of the coin. The other is that dullness and fatigue are important places to tolerate. Pretend mode, lack of vitality, may be the feelings that the patient needs the therapist to experience. As always, the challenge is a dilemma: when is dullness is called for and when is it unproductive?

There are also times when the feelings are too intensive, the playful aspects of the potential space are not possible to experience. The impact of the movie or book may be too strong; I cannot stand it. I have to close my eyes and say: "It's only on film, it's made up".

In her novel "The subtenant" Hanna Krall (1992) describes a visit to Majdanek by a woman called Maria. Maria's intention was to write "a new biography" for her father, who was murdered there. When she looks up at the ceiling in the barracks where the prisoners were gassed to death, she sees some bumps in the plaster. She thinks they are natural breaks in the mortar until she realizes that they are scratches made by the prisoners when they were suffocated to death. After this realization, fiction is not possible. There is no place for potential space in Majdanek. Memories and images of rape, assaults, and torture are hard to locate in the potential space.

The experience of the potential space is usually out of awareness, it is like the air we breathe, like water for the fish. We notice it when it disappears or when someone directs our attention to it. As we meet new people, and especially in relationships that are emotionally charged, we may reflect on the specific character of the relational space that emerges. When the relationship has found its forms, its character often becomes less visible.

An illustration:

The patient is extremely lonely; he has hardly any family, few friends, and work colleagues. Sometimes in the afternoon he goes to a pub, takes a beer, and looks around. He knows pretty well the people who come. Most of them come in groups, often from work as it seems. He has noticed some of the young women who seem to come right after work. The therapist has step by step become acquainted with the guests. The patient has various fantasies about them. There is a lady the patient thinks he would like to know, a couple of men he is envious of and several that he has negative opinions about. This group of persons becomes a gallery for feelings, fantasies, or thoughts. The therapist is invited to the patient's pub playground, to a world of potential contacts, romances, and dramas. They create shared images of possibilities. One day, the patient says that he was thrown out because he had been drunk and started fighting. The therapist realizes that she feels disappointed; she shared the pub world with the patient. The pub had become not only a place for taking a beer and looking around; it was a place to fantasize about, like the toys in play therapy with children.

The potential space is characterized by uncertainty. We must dare to let the therapy relationship evolve in its own tracks. If we know the end, it will be as pointless to remain in it as to see a film that has been spoiled to us. Mental health problems can be seen as expressions of lack of flexibility, of locks in the person's ability to explore alternative perspectives, of fear of uncertainty. Mental health is to be curious, open to new experiences. To promote experiences in the potential space experiences is to break the "it-is-what-it-is" feeling about the world (Gentile, 2007, p. 568).

The illustration shows that the therapeutic potential space, although based on the patient's experiences, is mutually created. When Ferenczi urged therapists to be open and authentic with their patients, one reason was to provide reparative relational experiences, a compensation for negative relationships with key figures, in line with later models of corrective emotional experiences (e.g. Alexander & French, 1946). The relational idea of openness and spontaneity is rather to fully participate in the creation of intersubjective space, to move to the intimate edge of the relationship (Ehrenberg, 1992), to be open to places where neither therapist not patient have been before.

David

Anne had thought for a while that David often looked bleak when he arrived. It used to change when they started talking, but Anne thought she would comment on it.

- I've noticed that you often seem gloomy when I see you in the waiting room. It usually changes when we start talking, but I thought I want to ask you about it.
- People say that I look angry.
- They do? I wouldn't say angry, but serious and a little bit downcast.
- Perhaps I get into a special mood when I'm seeing you. Somehow, I become more vulnerable.
- It's interesting that you say vulnerable. I've been thinking about how I react when you look like that. I feel that I should perhaps comfort you or take care of you in some way.
- That would feel odd to me. Not so many people are comforting me nowadays. Most people get angry at me.
- So what do you think about my feeling like that?
- Well, we have a special relationship. I thought about it last time I was here, that I kind of feel touched when I realize that you in some way understand what it's like for me.
- It seems as if you like it. I'm not that age, but it's as if I were your parent.
- A very unusual parent then. My experience is that parents take care of their own needs. I'd rather have you as an older sister. I've always longed for an older sister. Someone who could show me how to be as a grown-up. It feels like I'm never certain about what's right, what I should feel.
  Something in David's voice makes Anne feel quite touched. She has no siblings, but she has always longed for an older sister.
- So what would the sister do?
- Tell me how to live, what to appreciate, I think.
- You think I know that?

Although they enter the fantasy intentionally, they get engaged in it. The session continues with fantasies about what could have happened if they had been siblings.

How to do in practice?

Many parents have experienced the joy of inventing a story together with their child. "Once, the dad and the girl decided to go into the forest. The forest was dark and seemed dangerous. But the dad held the girl's hand".

The story line develops in its own ways. The child inserts new lines. The parent and the child may leave it unfinished to be continued the next day. Or they may tell it in a new form each time they tell it. The story is created during the process, but it is also "found", in their memories and experiences. They may be aware that the story has roots, but its vitality comes from their creativity.

A therapy illustration:

The work has mostly concerned the patient's avoidance of serious contacts with women, in part due to betrayals and disappointments. During several weeks, the patient has been ill, and the sessions have been cancelled. When the patient returns to therapy, the therapist asks whether the patient has missed the therapy. The patient does not express any strong engagement in the question.

- I thought about calling you, but I felt uncertain whether you would appreciate it.
- I don't know. I guess I would.
- It may sound odd, but I felt too much like a mother, and so I decided to abstain.
- I think I would have liked it. I feel a bit shy now that you say that.
- Shy for what?
- For your feelings about me. I didn't think you had such feelings.
- I didn't before, I kind of found them now.

The participants start exploring emotions that are not clear to any of them, that are created during the dialogue. They create conditions for the feelings to evolve.

The fact that the therapist contributes to the development of a potential space experience means that she may also initiate it in a way that she thinks fits the patient, in the same way as the parent may start a story with her child that she thinks is suitable.

In this case, the therapist knows that the patient has problems with letting someone bother about him. He may feel uncomfortable about the thought that someone might think about him. Others are preoccupied with worries that specific persons do not call, do not text, and do not think about them. The therapist's task is to present the opening, like the squiggle.

Framing the potential space

Potential space is not a pedagogic device, it is a way to understand a complex and sometimes scaring relational world. The significance of the teddy bear is due to the absence of the mother. The reason for authors to write novels may be to make unthinkable reality bearable. The potential space exists between the commonplace and the overwhelming.

There may be a need to frame the potential space, as it may be important to indicate that play is play. It may be important to make clear that it is a tentative and explorative attempt to understand challenging life situations.

An illustration:

The patient, who is between 50 and 60, was left by his wife some years ago. He became desolate and felt very lonesome. His wife's infidelity lowered his self-confidence. He started in therapy with a somewhat younger woman. Rather soon, he fell in love with her. He realized that they would never become a couple, but he could not abstain from walking the quarters where she lived, follow her on Facebook, trying to figure out how she lived. After some time, the therapist fell ill and had to stop the therapy. The patient was still depressed and had anxiety attacks. He is now in a new therapy with a therapist about his own age. He has started asking the therapist if she is married or separated, whether she has children, what part of the country she comes from. Although the questions seem harmless, the therapist is wary about answering. After reflecting on the situation, she realizes that it would be fruitful to use it.

– Recently, you have asked quite a lot about my private life, and I guess you have realized that I'm cautious about answering. I thought that I'd like to say something about it. I guess that you in some way ask what I think of you, whether I appreciate you, perhaps even if I might consider becoming friends with you.

– Well, I understand that you have a lot of friends. But I've had the fantasy that we might perhaps see each other when the therapy is over. I'm so uncertain whether anyone might really want to be with me and not only chat over the fence.

– I think it might be valuable if we try to talk about our feelings and fantasies about each other. I would like to start by saying that we will not be friends afterwards. That says nothing about whether we would like each other or not, it's just a device to make it possible to use our fantasies and dreams. So, let's think that we put kind of a frame around what we say, in order to know that this is a special mental place where we are as earnest as we may. What do you think of that?

By framing in this way, the therapist actively creates a common space where a special sort of mental sharing can take place. There is no guarantee for openness, but it creates an opportunity. It is like a theatre scene where all know that things may happen that are in some way outside the ordinary life. And like theatre, what happens within this frame becomes dull and dopey if it does not have a potential tie to reality.

Making the frame too visible may sometimes be felt as a way of down-playing the affective intensity, to play safe. But a formulated frame may make it possible to open for creative reflections. This might also make it easier for the therapist to dare approach difficult issues, like if the patient seems threatening or suicidal. In these situations, it may be important to actively and clearly state that what the therapist is going to say is in a purposefully created potential space, a room for reflections rather than statements.

Devices for framing

To put a frame around the potential space can be made explicitly as suggested earlier. But the therapist often uses more subtle linguistic devices to mark that the ongoing experience is in the potential space. Verb forms like the subjunctive mode may be useful: "We might think" or "If we were". Another device is "hedging", which means indicating that the statement is provisional or tentative (Lakoff, 1973; Oddli & Rønnestad, 2012) in order to obtain "hearer acceptance, avoidance of commitment and intentional vagueness" (Clemen, 1997, p. 239).

Making a self-disclosure may be an indication that the therapist wants to emphasize the special nature of the conversation. Self-disclosures can have the same role as "ostensive cues" (Allison & Fonagy, 2016), emphasizing that the therapist wants to say something important and special.

An example:
The patient has for several weeks evoked irritation in the therapist. The therapist has realized that such reactions seem to be common among persons in the patient's relational world. Would it be possible, and helpful, to express them?

– I'd like to talk about something that I have observed about my reactions in our contact for a while. You may have noticed it, but I am not sure. I have found that I feel irritated from time to time. I'm not always sure what the anger is about, but I often notice it when you talk about your partner. When I say this, how does it feel to you?

This formulation shows how the therapist puts her reaction in a semantic context intended to make it useful as material for reflection. The therapist steps outside her reaction and comments that it is an observation. "When I step outside myself and look into my mind, I find", the therapist tries to convey. The point with self-disclosures in this context is that the therapist demonstrates that she looks into her mind and shows that she tries to formulate something that has not been formulated before. Self-disclosure in this context is a way of disclosing the therapist's explorative intention.

The shared potential space

In therapy, potential space is intersubjectively created. It differs from the teddy bear and cultural experiences by developing in the intersubjective space, as a third.

An illustration:
When the patient describes his latest meeting with his child, the therapist associates to a dream that the patient related some time ago.

– When you talked about the feeling of loneliness that you had when you met your daughter, I was reminded about the dream you talked about. You know the dream about the boy who ran away, and you couldn't find him.

- Was that in a forest or ...? I'm not sure I remember.
- No, it was in a town. There was a house and the boy disappeared in the house.
- It was in a big house, wasn't it?
- As I remember it, it was a small and tall house. And the boys ran up the stairs and you were afraid he would fall down. I thought of that dream when you talked about your daughter. The fear of abandonment.

Who is the dreamer, who's inner world is it? The coalescence of the patient's and the therapist's fantasies and images create a shared potential space. The therapist might have remained silent, does invade the patient's mental space, or contributes to the shared space, with something that had stayed in her mind.

17 Listen for conflicts, stay in conflicts

The tool

In meaningful therapy, the participants engage in the therapeutic interaction with experiences, expectations, engagements, values, and needs. Conflicts in interactions are ubiquitous. Even though we normally try to agree and gloss over disagreements, meticulous studies of dialogues in therapy and elsewhere show that we seldom succeed (Viklund, Holmqvist, & Zetterqvist Nelson, 2009). We rather disagree about most things: what we experience together, what significance the experiences may have, and what we should do about problems that arise.

Usually, conflicts are so insignificant that we do not notice them, and we do not care about them. In relational therapy, however, we try to attend to them. The tool is to listen for conflicts, to try to become aware of them, and to reflect on whether they should be brought up in the conversation. It is not a matter of bringing them up just for the sake of it, but to use their potential therapeutic value. When the conflict has become visible, when both the therapist and the patient know that they are in it, it is up to the therapist to think: "Now, now we are there, now we are working". Take a deep breath, enter the conflict, enjoy it or fear it, but stay in it!

The purpose

Human interaction is to a great extent about managing conflicts. They can be subtle ("When I started talking about my children, I got the feeling that you looked away and got something else in mind, but I may be mistaken") or obvious ("If we want to understand your problems, you can't just blame others for them"). We develop as relational beings by dealing with conflicts. There are, of course, different cultural and personal rules and frameworks for how conflicts are handled. In Japan, conflicts are handled in a different way than on Manhattan. But in all human contexts, dealing with conflicts advance personal development. By being clear with her clues and

DOI: 10.4324/9781003026914-17

observations, the therapist enables the patient and herself to become aware of and learn to manage conflicts, to recognize feelings in herself and the patient, to be curious about what she wants and what the patient wants. Conflicts clarify how we feel about each other and make it possible to find new ways of being together.

The dilemma

Meeting the patient authentically involves risks. If we go back to the tennis metaphor, tennis players can agree to play easy balls. It may be nice for a while. But such play never engages. No one feels lost, no one gets angry or shameful or happy. In nice play, there is time to think before the ball comes. The players can be careful about their initiatives, avoid challenging in a way that could be felt as offensive.

Psychotherapy can also be nice. Therapist and patient can avoid challenging each other. But then, there will be no match. In engaged therapy, the therapist endeavours to create a dialogue where she is as vulnerable as the patient because the topics are emotionally charged, vital, and decisive – the direction uncertain.

Principles

Relational treatment is based on a conflict perspective. In contrast to traditional psychoanalytic theory, the conflict is not primarily intrapsychic; it is first and foremost interpersonal, between patient and therapist. This view does not detract from the knowledge that persons have intrapsychic conflicts. The idea is rather pragmatic: when the conflict takes shape between the therapist and the patient, it becomes possible to deal with in a way that is constructive for the patient. An illustration:

The therapist has for some time been annoyed that the patient uses something that smells during the session and that stays in the room when he has gone. Maybe perfume, maybe shaving water. A few times the therapist has been forced to apologize to the next patient for the smell although she has opened the window.

The situation could be interpreted as indicating that the patient uses perfume because he is afraid of smelling bad, perhaps without being fully aware of it. Or he may want to make himself attractive to the therapist. A psychoanalytic interpretation might be that he wants to stay in the room with the therapist with his scent, in some sense invading her room. Or maybe even take possession of her room and protect himself from that thought by perfuming it.

The relational therapist tells the patient that she has noticed the scent.

–   Yes, it's probably my shaving water. Do you think it smells too much?

- I have actually reacted to it on several occasions. I felt uncertain whether to say anything to you about it. It does embarrass me as I think someone else coming in might sense it.
- That's really embarrassing! You could have said that before.
- That's true. In fact, I hadn't decided how annoyed I felt so I didn't know what to say before. And to be honest, I was also afraid of hurting you.

The therapist could have just asked the patient not to put on the perfume next time. She chooses to give a rather full explanation of her motives in order to remain in the potential conflict.

- You could have said it earlier. If you had told me, I would of course have stopped using it. I hope you're not just trying to be kind to me when you sound like you didn't know what to think.
- Of course, I should have said it earlier. Maybe I was unnecessarily careful. I hear you get disappointed.
- I feel ashamed because I have put you in a difficult situation.
- So, my hesitation put you in a worse situation than if I had told you at once.
- Sometimes I think you're not as tough on me as I need. You don't need to be careful about me.

The therapist tells the patient about her conflict about communicating. This makes it possible to open for a more intense interaction than just a question about the reasons to use it or a plea to avoid it. Interpersonal conflict is invited.

To strengthen and to challenge the relationship

Therapy is based on a collaborative relationship between therapist and patient. Different schools have different methods for strengthening the alliance. Some schools use education, other approaches underline that fast results promote the alliance (Foa, Hembree, Rothbaum, & Rach, 2019).

Relational therapy is paradoxical in the sense that it, while basically trying to increase the patient's confidence in the therapy process, also challenges the therapeutic relationship. A simple example:

The patient is a 28-year-old man who lives alone. He wants help for his feelings of loneliness and anxiety. He has some friends, mostly male. Over the years, he has had some shorter relationships with women, but he has never lived with anyone. He does not have any plans to establish a stable relationship and has no longing for children. He has the friends he needs, and his sexual needs are satisfied with the women he sleeps with now and then.

The therapist thinks the patient has problems with emotional closeness. He seems to keep his contacts at a distance, and he does not become dependent on anyone. Although the patient has a kind manner, it is hard to know what he thinks about the treatment. Occasionally, the therapist raises the question about how close the patient comes to male and female friends, how intimate they become, if he longs for closer friends, if he can feel vulnerable with any of them.

– So, you met the woman you dated before.
– Yes, we spent the night together. She is nice.
– Would you say there is a touch of love in it?
– No. I'm not ready for that, I think.
– So, what happens?
– We enjoy it both of us.
– You know, I find it hard to really get at what you feel. Could you help me?
– Your model is simple but faulty. You think I need a stable relationship. I don't. I get fed up with your ideas about confidentiality and closeness.
– You seem annoyed when I try to challenge your ways of being with friends and partners. I wonder if that brings us apart.
– It's ok that you challenge me. We have a professional relationship, don't we? I pay you for provoking me, that's fine.
– It doesn't sound very confidential to me. It sounds like a staged battle. That's not my picture of what we're doing.

The therapist raises a relevant question. She could have waited until the patient brought it up. But she chooses to go at the issue of closeness in the relationship. The patient's reactions make it possible to bring the issue of closeness into the relationship with the therapist.

Empathy

Therapist empathy is a facilitative stance for patient change. It needs a process to arise, it usually does not come off immediately, in contrast to other reactions. When the patient shares a hideous experience, the therapist may become emotionally overwhelmed, she may feel sympathy for him, she may have a wish to console. But empathy is more complicated. It comes from a process of trying on, being wrong, trying again, successively entering the patient's world – and again finding that she did not truly understand. Empathy evolves from negotiating.

– It must feel awful to you that your mother has been diagnosed with dementia at her early age.
– That's ok in some way. I know it may be seen as unfair. Most persons my age have healthy parents. But it is as it is.
– Sometimes people get unreasonably angry at persons who do not have the same hard experiences as you yourself.

- I don't get angry. I think I give up. It feels hopeless.
- You mean the possibilities to cure her?
- No, I mean that I won't be able to talk with her anymore. Soon, she will not recognize me.
- So you will feel alone.
- Yes, I share a lot with my mom. She knows most about me. It's almost like we're best friends.
- But you have your wife?
- That's different. My mom has known me all my life, she knows most about me.
- Even things about your wife?
- Some of them, yes. You may think it sounds strange, and my wife is sometimes angry at me about it. In some way, I'll lose myself when my mother becomes dement.
- It's true that one's mother is the person who has known you for the longest time. You will not be able to ask how you were as a child.
- That's not the thing. The thing is that she knows how to comfort me. When I become desolate, it's only mom who can solace me.

The therapist tries actively to understand the significance of the relation with the mother. By asking and comparing with her own experiences, the understanding increases. The empathy process evolves in the combination of own experiences and ideas, questions, and unexpected answers. The empathy process is a telling illustration of subtle continuous conflict resolution in therapy.

Therapy complications

Empirical studies have repeatedly found that positive therapist in-session affects are associated with symptom reduction (Chui, Hill, Kline, Kuo, & Mohr, 2016). Negative countertransference reactions have been found to lead to worsened patient reactions (Hayes, Gelso, & Hummel, 2011). However, this is a static view of the therapist's stance, basically implying that the therapist is seen as delivering facilitative conditions for patient change. In a relational perspective, negative countertransference is a chance, an opportunity for mutual reflection.

In a study of negative therapist countertransference, rated after the session, and symptom change the next session, Falkenström & Holmqvist (2021) found that in BRT, more negative reactions were associated with less symptoms. A possible reason could be that disclosure and active use of countertransference reactions opened for mentalizing about the therapeutic situation, probably strengthened by perceived genuineness in the therapist.

Although good and constructive relationships are built on positive and genuine feelings, on openness and mutual understanding, they may also contain tensions, disagreements, deadlocks, hassles, squabbles. A vital relationship thrives from fluctuations between intimacy, openness, and acceptance on one hand, and distance, disappointment, and anger on the other. Continuous distance would be devastating, of course, but so would permanent closeness.

In the relational literature, the concept of ruptures in the relationship is a key idea. Sometimes, ruptures are easily detectable. But the concept's usefulness is related to its focus on subtle variants of misunderstandings, mismatches, hurdles in the relationship.

Safran and Muran (2000) described two types of alliance ruptures: confrontation and withdrawal. They also presented a model, based on task analyses of therapeutic dialogues, for strategies to resolve the ruptures. The strategies delineated by Safran and Muran clearly point to the epistemological dilemma that relational theory grapples with. On one hand, the therapist identifies relational trouble that can be understood as an expression of the patient's previous relational propensities. On the other, she knows that the problem is mutual, a shared enactment (Benjamin, 2017), influenced by the therapist's proclivities and by the ongoing interaction (Muran, 2019). Epistemologically, the model points to the tension between positivistic and constructionistic perspectives.

David

During the Christmas holidays, David calls his therapist to ask for an extra session. Anne decides that as she has nothing planned, it is ok for her. When he comes, he tells her that he has been drunk for three days. Anne is surprised; she did not think that drinking was a problem at this time. His wife is extremely upset and accuses him for not taking his alcoholism seriously. He has been rude to both her and the children. Now, he is remorseful.

– How did it start?
– I was just fed up with everything. I'm not getting any better. So I wanted to cheer myself up as it was Christmas.
– So you were fed up with our work too?
– In a way, yes. I don't feel any better now than I did when we started.
– So you're angry?
– It's hard to tell you. You're kind and I think you really want to help me. But it doesn't help much.
– So what did you think when you bought your beers?
– That I will stop treatment, get an apartment of my own and start working at the garage.
  Anne becomes disappointed. She thinks he could have told her before.
– I wonder why you didn't tell me.
– You're so dedicated. I didn't want to disappoint you.
– But you did. I do feel disappointed that you didn't talk about your feelings before.

- Shame on me! I'm always a failure. I try my best, I thought I was kind to you.

By admitting that she was disappointed, Anne opens for a conflict between them. From David's side, it is a confrontative rupture. Before trying to resolve it, Anne is keen to make it clear between them. The session continues with talk about their feelings and expectations for each other. The dialogue could be understood as an externalization of David's ambivalence about handling things on his own and relying on Anne. Relationally, Anne's reaction is also influenced by her own history; in addition, the specific nature of the conflict is coloured by its own process.

How to do in practice

Conflicts are essential in the development of the ability to negotiate roles, wishes, expectations (Tronick, 1998). The nature of the interaction becomes visible when it becomes entangled, messy; when the conversation does not flow on and the words do not hook into each other, when one feels baffled, provoked, or questioned. Or maybe one of the participants just does not understand the other, and wonders what he or she is really thinking and what to say about it.

Interaction skills develop in the unplanned relational skills exercises that a whole life's relationships offer. Sometimes, we learn new things about ourselves in relationships, often we just continue falling in the same traps time and again. The point of relational therapy is to open for new relational learning, for new understanding, new ways of relating.

Psychotherapy is based on collaboration about treatment goals and procedures to achieve them. As a treatment, psychotherapy is special in the sense that it is often an open question how the goal should be specified and the best way to get there. Several models have been developed that discuss how goals and tasks are negotiated (Fonagy, Luyten, & Allison, 2015; Frank & Frank, 1993).

Negotiations around the mutual work can end up in enactments and alliance ruptures. Enactment is the relational equivalent of resistance. Resistance is usually not consciously experienced as such; the same pertains to enactments. They may be sensed as problematic situations, hard to explore, hard to get on from.

Confrontational ruptures are usually visible to the participants. But most ruptures are of the withdrawal type. It takes some time to become aware that the conversation is not productive or vital, takes place in a pretend type of way, or has ended up within narrow limits or in a constrained mode.

Although the alliance rupture-resolution model usually presupposes that the patient causes the alliance break, many studies have shown that ruptures are often caused by the therapist, sometimes by design, sometimes unwittingly (Muran & Eubanks, 2020).

An illustration:

The patient is pessimistic in general and particularly about his job. He thinks he has to leave it because he does not like to work in a team. The therapist has tried to encourage him to talk with his boss, to no avail. She has tried to stimulate him to find friends, without much success. She has talked about her frustration, about hesitance to engage in the therapy from the patient's side. The patient does not oppose, he feels nothing will help her. The therapist reflects on other ways she could have used. She could have been more empathic, or more encouraging. She is now ready to give up, she thinks that she cannot help him.

The therapy seems to be a failure. But she hesitates to make the patient disappointed. She fears he will have guilt feelings, that the therapy will be a new piece on his stack of failures.

In this situation, material in the form of an enactment has emerged. The therapist did not make it happen; it was no intervention. It was genuine therapeutic work that landed in a situation with hopelessness. The therapist's self-disclosure about disappointment will not be an uncommitted comment, it will be a genuine and engaged statement about her feelings about their mutual work. The therapist will recognize her part in the failure, but not as a therapeutic contrivance.

The rupture-repair model suggests that the therapist, by exploring the rupture together with the patient, may help him access previously disavowed emotional positions. In the confrontative rupture, the patient, ideally, becomes aware of his vulnerability and need for support; the withdrawing patient, hopefully, becomes able to express his assertiveness.

Although useful for pedagogical and theoretical reasons, the idea that patient characteristics may be discerned in rupture patterns is questionable on epistemological grounds. Ruptures are mutually created. It is, of course, feasible and sometimes meaningful to chisel out the contributions of the partners and work with these problems as individual patterns. The relational perspective implies, however, a more dyadic view of the therapeutic process, where not only contributions come from both partners but also the very process engenders its own problems.

There may be an idealized idea of quarrels that clean the air, followed by reunion and good feelings. This is sometimes true, especially for the big ones. But more often, the resolution of one mismatch leads over to the next. It is like walking on the tussocks on a moor, one tussock that sinks into water is followed by the next.

Should we attend to all these? Of course not, it would be a compulsive terror. Most of them are observable on frames of video-films or in detailed transcriptions but not in the mind of the participants. It is a relational skill, a sensitivity to the situation, to know when to acknowledge that something in the communication seems to squeak.

Sometimes, the conflict becomes more or less conscious to the participants but is left behind. But more often, it is solved in the moment, perhaps without conscious attention. If it is noticed, patient and therapist may talk about how they perceive it, perhaps leading to perceptions of new aspects of the relationship. Or, when in affect, they may say less well-thought-out things to each other and hopefully reconcile later.

Conflicts may seem new when they occur, but it is an understandable therapist reaction to try to find patterns in them (Luborsky, 1984), both in the patient and in herself. A challenge in relational therapy is to be responsive to new aspects of the conflict; to see how, although influenced by old patterns, it has twisted slightly, as in a kaleidoscope. It is like in a marriage: you might tend to see the same conflict coming up again and try to avoid it. Or you may see indications of new aspects in the conflict, attend to them and develop.

Becoming part of the conflict

Many therapy schools propose that the therapist should not show her emotional engagement too openly. Reactions that can be held back and where the usefulness of disclosing them is not obvious should remain in the mind of the therapist. Relational therapists use their engagement in a more active way. Some examples:

> The patient describes problematic behavior: he is often on sick leave, he says that he is abusive towards his wife, drinks too much, quarrels with friends. The therapist feels uncertain about the situation. She is upset but she also suspects that the patient exaggerates. She tells him about her worries as well as about her skepticism. The patient becomes hurt about her suspicion. She tries to explain but has difficulties finding the right words.

> The patient feels lonely and abandoned. The therapist has warm feelings for him and decides to tell him. The patient feels belittled. The therapist tries to clarify but the patient apparently hates getting sympathy.

The illustrations show how active therapists often get trapped into problematic situations. Imagine a boxing match. The boxers punch each other and protect themselves from the punches of the other. When they are a bit distant from each other, they can move back and forth, punch and jump. But sometimes they get into a clinch. They come so close that no one can punch. No one dares to go back because the other will take the chance. Instead, they lock each other with arms and gloves. The judge has to break. She separates them, sets them apart and urges them to start boxing again.

In relational therapy, the clinch is the enactment. Patient and therapist get stuck in each other emotionally. They cannot move. The active therapist stance may beget conflicts. The conflict is not planned, it is a potential consequence of the therapist's engagement.

If the conceptualization of the patient's problems is too narrow, if the template for what is to be done is too rigid, the patient will not become visible. If the therapist locks the patient into an action plan too quickly, she will not know who the patient is. The therapist who is too formal and rigid about making plans will protect herself from being entrapped.

18 Meta-communication

The tool

Meta-communicating means talking about communication, standing next to it, and commenting on it. Meta is a Greek word meaning about, over and after. Meta-communication is thus communication about, over or after the communication. One of the basic human abilities, and where she differs from all other mammals, is her ability to see herself from the outside using language. Language allows us to comment on what we are talking about, on what happens between us.

Meta-communication is the essence of relational therapy. The material created in the interaction is used when therapists and patients meta-communicate with each other about how they talk with each other and how they react emotionally towards each other. It goes without saying that they need to talk about something else before they can talk about their conversation.

A parable could be the situation when the conversation is recorded. After a while you stop the camera, and then you look at what you did during the last minutes. "Do you see how I look at you there, I think I look sad". "Yes, you actually look sad, but I think that you may have been ashamed". "Yes, perhaps but I did not understand it, all the time I was occupied by my feeling that you would start crying".

Starting a meta-communication, thus shifting focus from the actual talk about the problem at hand or the patient's life situation to the relationship between the therapist and the patient requires judgement, empathy, courage, and purposeful awareness. It is important to do it with a sense for opportunity, relevance, and commitment, and for the patient's ability and motivation. To comment on the ongoing relationship can be made on a scale from a glance or a gesture to a detailed description. Once you have started to meta-communicate, it is important to be sensitive about how long it is fruitful to hold on to it and when to return to other themes. The driving force in meta-communication should always be the emotional urgency.

DOI: 10.4324/9781003026914-18

The purpose

The purpose of meta-communication is to utilize the emotional interaction between therapist and patient to widen the possible ways of understanding relations. This very general description can accommodate everything from the therapist announcing that she tries to understand what the patient feels to inviting to a nuanced reflection on how it feels to talk about a trauma that the patient has experienced and the therapist perhaps fears hearing more about. Meta-communicating is a way to clarify the ongoing work. When reflecting about where the process is heading, it is important to continuously open for reconsiderations. To meta-communicate can be as simple as saying "Sometimes I get the feeling that we are grappling about the right way to go" or as delicate as trying to formulate subtle feelings of erotic longing, tenderness, or contempt that have arisen in the interaction.

The dilemma

Meta-communication is a technique. The therapeutic skill is to find occasions when it is appropriate to talk about the relationship. However, it would feel odd to think about technique in situations when we mutually struggle to understand emotionally sensitive situations, perhaps with the intention to understand the degree of intimacy between us. Meta-communicating about such issues is one of the most meaningful and compliacetd human activities we know. We do not exercise it. Studies of interaction between children and parents indicate that parents' ability to see and comment on the relationship with the child "from the outside" contributes to the child's mentalizing ability. The concept of "marked response" means that the parent is both empathic with the child and cognizant of the difference in relational position. But the parent does not train to provide marked responses. She may strive to understand the child, she may practise talking friendly. But she will hardly train being spontaneously worried in a way that is both authentic and at the same time shows the child that she can tolerate it. There is a fine line between practiced responsiveness and genuine, spontaneous curiosity about what is going on.

Principles

Humans can think about their own thoughts and about what their behaviour may mean for others. Other mammals can do many things that previously were seen as unique for homo sapiens. Apes can figure out what other individuals may think, crows can plan ahead of their actions. But only humans can say: "It strikes me that I may have sounded angry. I think I reacted to something in your voice without really becoming aware of it".

The two-level process

It is fascinating to look at sheep giving birth to their lambs. The lambs stand up almost immediately and start eating from the ewe. They have no idea of what they do. They have no plan, no conscious intention, no fear of something going wrong. Everything is driven by instinct, by the genetic program. If the ewe does not accept her lamb, is it reasonable to get angry at her? Yes, unreasonably. But with my reason, I understand that she has no intention. Sheep are not mean.

Parents, on the other hand, can be mean when they do not care for their babies. There may be reasons for the behaviour, but we feel that we have a right to place responsibility on the parent. Parents can reflect on their parenthood. They can mentally step outside themselves.

It is the parent's thinking and feeling about the relationship with the baby and my thinking and feeling about that relationship that makes us human. Usually, parent and child interactions float on. They enjoy the tenderness and warmth. They are in the midst of their feeling, "immersed" in it. But sometimes, for a moment or for a longer time, they think about their relationship. The milk does not come as it should. "What's wrong with me?" The parent feels an ounce of discomfort with the child. "Why do I think so?" The father does not think the mother is as beautiful as everyone says that new moms are. "Am I allowed to think so?".

The capacity to think about our thinking, our reactions, and to talk about them lie at the heart of human problems and human possibilities.

It is obvious that patients do not start therapy because they want to talk about the relationship with their therapist. They have problems or difficulties in their lives that they want to get help with. There are, in all therapies, occasions when the therapist must talk about the relationship with the patient. If the patient does not come, does not want to talk about his problems, or is openly critical of the therapist, it is necessary to talk about collaboration problems.

An illustration:

The young man recently made a serious suicide attempt: he wrote a farewell letter, arranged a snare to hang himself but changed his mind when he had his head in the snare. In the session, however, he prefers to talk about hiccups and hassles between himself and his friends. The therapist feels irritated as she knows that he was at the psychiatric emergency room a few days ago after the suicide attempt. The therapist thinks that the patient is in a kind of pretend bubble. At home, he seems to play with his daughter as usual.

– Although you have difficulties with your friends, I think we should talk about your suicide attempt.
– That was several days ago. I don't think of it any longer. And, in fact, it had to do with my best friend. I didn't feel appreciated by him any longer and that made me furious.

- What about your daughter? Did you think of her?
- You don't think I bother about her? You want me to have bad conscience?
- That's not my point. What I wonder is why we don't talk about your suicide attempt.
- I want to look forward. Do you want me to promise never to make an attempt? So we can leave it?
- I wonder what happens now. I want to talk about your suicide attempt, you don't. We get stuck. How do you look upon our talk?
- I think you exaggerate it. I never meant to.
- Ok. I take that. I may be stubborn.
- I think you are. But a realize that it seems funny that I won't say anything about it although I was at the hospital a few days ago.

This is a simple illustration of how the therapist tries to lift their eyes away from a pending clinch. We think about how we talk when it does not move on. Usually, we are in the middle of feeling. But often, recurrently, we stop and reflect. To "meta-think" and "meta-talk" was not invented as a treatment technique. We have done this since we evolved from homo habilis to homo sapiens. From the mere doing to also thinking, reflecting. When we communicate with each other, we move between being in the middle of the experience and seeing it from the outside, thinking about it and talking about it.

Meta-communication moves between being quite subtle and very explicit. It can also move between a more obvious technical measure ("I think we have to consider what just transpired between us") to a slight indication of awareness of the current emotional situation.

David

David has met an old friend in the town. They do not meet often, and the friend did not know that David was on sick leave. David did not tell him although their conversation touched the topic. Anne has reacted previously when David has avoided talking about his sick leave, for example, with parents at the swimming school. Anne thinks that he avoids the shame that he must confront if he tells them.

- Did you lie to your friend?
- Well I said it was good at work when he asked. It is good at work even though I am not there right now.
- So you avoided the truth?
- Do I always have to tell the truth? We don't know each other that well anymore. How would I benefit from having it spread out everywhere?
- I think it's good for you to talk about your situation frankly. I think your shame about it might dissipate.

– There is no one who is as aware of the shame as I am myself. I think I'm full of shame. Is that some kind of recipe, getting shamed by everyone? *Anne thinks about in what way it would help David to tell his friends about his sick leave. She thinks it may be part of David's difficulty in showing his vulnerability.*

– Well, I don't think you must tell everyone. But still I wonder. Could it be because you're a man that you don't want to show your vulnerability?

– Would that make any difference? That sounds old-fashioned. Like you're trying to put a label on me.
Anne feels a little bit ashamed. He might be right, perhaps she has prejudices about men. This does not seem to be the right track for the conversation.

– How did we end up here? You didn't want to talk about your sick leave with your friend and when I think about it, I'm not sure how relevant it would have been to do so. Perhaps I had preconceived notions that it's good for you to talk about your illness with all sorts of people and I might even end up in prejudices about men and women and become far too square.
Anne leaves the space open for David's reactions.

– ometimes you try to persuade me to things that I don't think are constructive. But you have seen how I avoid talking about it even with people where it would be reasonable. It's no wonder you thought I should have told my friend.

– No, you are right, but it feels like a lesson to me. Perhaps it's even hard for me to think that you may be vulnerable.

Anne backs from her line and instead invites them together to reflect on how they talk with each other. The invitation begins with her thinking about in which wheel tracks she herself has ended up.

How to do in practice?

The ways of commenting an ongoing relational interaction are endless. The same situation may evoke many different thoughts and feelings. Thoughts and feelings about an ongoing situation are contextualized; they are born from the wishes, hopes, and fears that have become actualized by the interaction and the expectations about what will happen.

To meta-communicate is not to make a statement at a seminar, it is to take a step on weak ice. Sometimes, the therapist wants to be certain, to make the meta-communication without any risk. Doing that, the meta-communication can become too intellectual, too abstract. It can easily become pretend mode-talk. It is important to follow the affective track. If the patient and therapist turn and twist what has been said just for the sake of it, they are in the pretend mode. With some exaggeration, what is said to the patient should be said with heart palpitation and nerves on the outside. The feeling should be: "It's now or never". or "If I don't say it now, I will regret it".

A good way to start meta-communicating is to *self-disclose*. The therapist can say: "I feel that my shoulders became tense. I guess that's some kind of feeling I have about our talk" instead of the patient-oriented "Can you feel what's in your shoulders?"

How often should the therapist comment on the relationship? The change of focus from the ongoing work to what is happening in the interaction should not be made on routine, it should be felt as urgent. The patient should be engaged in it, and the topic being addressed should remain in focus for some time. It is a balancing between the therapist's ability to make the patient understand that what is being addressed is important and not to insist if it is obvious that the patient does not become engaged.

Meta-communicating is no "Swiss army knife" for all purposes. In particular, it should not be a way of avoiding direct talk about problematic issues.

"The older patient disclosed that he did not sleep with his partner since several years. The young female therapist tried to ask for details, but the patient avoided such questions. The therapist had the choice between continuing asking about details and commenting on their interaction".

In this situation, a retreat to meta-communicating about the patient's and the therapist's shyness about exchanging details about the patient's attempts to renew his sexual life might be constructive, but it could also be a way of evading challenging questions about details in the patient's life.

Finding the right moment

The patient grew up in a family of violence. His father beat his mother, and sometimes he struck the patient. In his current life with a partner, he was prone to get outburst, but he never became physically violent. The therapy had focused on his traumatic memories and on his present explosive temper. During the last sessions, the therapist had become more and more frustrated by the patient's insistence on his way of describing his outbursts. He admitted that he could become angry, often without reason. But when he talked about the situations when he became threatening, he usually found reasons in the other's behaviour. The therapist had several times thought she would disclose her frustration but every time she had hesitated as she thought he had a need to express his anger at people.

– You know my wife never lets me finish talking. I get extremely frustrated and sometimes quite angry. No wonder, I think. She can be quite interruptive when I try to tell her about my problems at work. I guess she is envious about me having an interesting work. In any case, show ought to listen to me when she understands that what I'm saying is important to me. I don't think she has a right to stop me.

- What do you mean, not a right?
- To me, living together means that partners are interested in each other. My wife isn't.

The therapist realizes that she is getting annoyed again at the self-righteousness of her patient. Now, she thinks is an occasion for talking about it.

- I want to talk with you about something that I've thought of from time to time, or felt, perhaps I should say. You may feel hurt, but I think it can be useful if we talk about it. Sometimes when you talk about the reasons for you getting upset and angry, I get quite frustrated and sometimes irritated. I'm not certain why but it may be the tone that you use when talking about persons like now when you talked about your wife.

The therapist has avoided this occasion. She could have rounded her irritation and talked about her patient's anger and how he might express it in other ways.

Remaining silent or meta-communicating?

Imagine a father doing the dishes when the child comes homes. She sits down at the table and starts talking about everyday things. Eventually, she begins to talk about some problematic relations with peers. The father tries to ask but the daughter becomes silent. After a while she says a few things. The father makes some comments, and the daughter gets really irritated.

- Why are you always so curious?
- I thought you wanted me to know.
- You always misunderstand everything. You don't know how it is in schools nowadays.

Should the father comment on their conversation? He just tried to understand. He realizes that the subject is sensitive, that the daughter wants to tell but in her own way.

In therapy, a similar situation can be handled by silence from the therapist. Or by renewed questions. Or by talking about her reactions without requiring an answer from the patient.

Practical tips

There are situations when meta-communication comes of its own. But sometimes the therapist has to be pedagogical, she has to describe how and why it may be important to think about the relationship. Here are some tips about how to introduce it:

- Tell the patient to imagine that you have played in a film and now you want to look at it.
- Suggest that you use your recent interaction as a projective picture, open for diverse fantasies
- Be mindful about the balance between being too concrete (psychic equivalence; "You said this and then I said that") and only fantasy (pretend mode; "I could have said any odd thing as it is only therapy").

19 Model mentalizing

The tool

Two tasks are central in relational therapy: to engage in attempts to understand the patient's current problems with curiosity and engagement, and to attend to the ongoing interaction, looking for reflection opportunities. It is to be mindful-in-action (Safran & Muran, 2000), to "get involved while paying attention" (Seligman, 2014, p. 649).

Reflecting on the ongoing interaction is the basic way to enhance mentalizing. Time and again, therapist and patient lose their reflective stance, as do all participants in engaging interactions. There are moments in life when explicit mentalizing is the wrong thing to do. But often, mentalizing is the tool for tolerating and understanding the immediate interaction. In the therapeutic interaction, not only the patient but also the therapist loses this mental capacity. Recognition of such failures are key moments for modelling mentalizing. By reflecting on what is happening and what feelings have been aroused, the therapist shows that she is open to the patient's understanding as well as her own, that the interaction can be understood in different ways and that full understanding is seldom attainable. An important part of the work is for the therapist to identify her own difficulties in mentalizing and, when she becomes aware of them, to share the discovery with the patient (Fonagy, Gergely, Jurist, & Target, 2002).

Mentalizing is mostly implicit. It unfolds without conscious attention; it is a relational autopilot. It becomes a therapeutic tool when we pay attention to it, when we discover it or realize that we lost it.

The purpose

Mentalizing is born together with other persons. Children develop their mentalizing ability primarily in interaction with adults they trust. In treatment, mentalizing takes place together with a therapist whom the patient has confidence in. The therapeutic relationship is fertile soil for mentalizing. A way for the therapist to contribute to its fertility is to openly mentalize, to disclose and invite to reflections about her own reactions, ponderings,

DOI: 10.4324/9781003026914-19

hunches. And to attend as best she can to non-mentalizing periods in the communication.

The dilemma

The goal of treatment is rarely to improve mentalization. But mentalizing is probably an important change mechanism in many therapy methods (Allison & Fonagy, 2016; Markowitz, Milrod, Luyten, & Holmqvist, 2019). The ability to understand and cope with the complexities of our own and our fellow human's emotional reactions is an important prerequisite for us to feel secure with each other and to face life's challenges. When the impulse-driven or depressed person only sees one explanation of what happened between him and another person, only is aware of a small range of feelings, improved mentalizing may be a main therapeutic goal.

There are situations where mentalizing is an obstacle. When the patient exposes himself to anxiety-provoking situations, when he has finally contact with pure rage towards the person who maltreated him, mentalizing should stay behind.

Therapy moves between security and uncertainty as does life. The lover responding to his girlfriend's question: "Do you love me?" with an overly mentalizing and reflecting response does not pass the test. But when they start quarrelling, implicit as well as explicit mentalizing are useful.

The principles

People are curious about each other's minds. We learn about ourselves by trying to figure out how other people think and feel. In orthodox psycho-analysis, the patient's curiosity about the therapist is turned back to himself: "It seems as if you think I don't care about you. I wonder if anything comes to your mind when you feel that".

In relational work, the therapist might say: "I've thought about in what way I care about you. Sometimes I get the impression that you think I don't, and I've realized it disturbs me. What do you think of that?", directing the focus rather to the interaction. The material to reflect on is sought in mutual experiences rather than only in the patient's thoughts and fantasies.

Mentalizing is a trait-based but situationally influenced capacity, in many ways similar to a person's ability to tolerate conflicting mental representa-tions (Fonagy, Edgcumbe, Moran, Kennedy, & Target, 1993). However, this description mainly pertains to explicit mentalizing. Implicit mentalizing, relational knowledge online, is about process, about intuitive understanding of situations and competence to handle continuously emerging challenges.

The relation between explicit, conscious, sometimes verbally formulated mentalizing, and implicit, process-oriented implicit mentalizing is poorly studied. Although establishing a mental distance between immediate thoughts and feelings and reflections about them is important for our ability to deal with mental health problems, it is uncertain to what extent such reflection is important for ongoing procedural knowing. Mental problems can often be described as lack of distance between the subject and his experiences, as thoughts and feelings that get stuck in us, bite into us, do not let go. When anxiety thoughts do not let go, we cannot sleep; when we are certain that the body has a deadly disease, we are in the grips of hypochondria.

Shared uncertainty and curiosity about how the interaction between patient and therapist should be understood, where it is heading, what the participants may sense about the other's intentions and feelings, is the way to improve mentalizing.

David

David and Anne had decided that they should talk about David's experiences in childhood as they might have significance for his feelings of loneliness and alienation. David liked to talk about his childhood and Anne was often touched by his stories. When they started, she tried to help David tell more details about his experiences, and to stay in the feelings that they evoked. Anne thought they made constructive work around his experiences of loneliness and abandonment. David talked about his anger at his mother, of his shame in front of his classmates. He remembered that he had been quite scared about the possibility that his mother might disappear. By and by, however, Anne had felt less and less engaged in these stories. It took some time before she realized it, as David was a good narrator and often was emotionally affected when telling them. During his recounting, Anne used to feel that something important was taking place. Afterwards, however, she often felt that the therapy had not moved ahead. One day when she had listened to a new story about how David had been left by his cousins, she had a very distinct feeling that although David was quite upset about his memories, it was in some way therapeutically futile.

–   I do realize that this was hard for you. But I want to share another feeling. Despite the pain that these memories evoke in you, I realize that I'm not quite as engaged as I'd thought I'd be. I feel a little bit as if there were a filter between what you say and what I feel.
–   So, you mean that my stories bore you?
–   No, that's not what I mean. It's much more subtle. I do really get touched. Perhaps I try to say that there's a gap between my expectation of feelings and the feelings that I do experience. It's like you listen to a story that's important for the storyteller but you get the feeling that it has been told a number of times before. I don't think that you've told this story before but still I get that kind of feeling.
–   I think I know what you're talking about. Sometimes I have the feeling that you don't listen in the same way as before, or at least do not react in the same way.

- It's like your telling in some way doesn't get into gear, like we're going at idle. Like we're going back into the same wheel tracks again and again.
  ... (pause)
- I must say that I feel quite sad and a bit offended by what you say. I'm trying to come to grips with my feelings of loneliness and I think they have roots in my childhood situation.
- So, you're disappointed at me? Or?
- I think I feel that you in some way dismiss me, like you don't think I'm interesting anymore.
- Ok, yes, I realize that in some sense you may feel that I abandon you emotionally. Like I'm leaving you with your memories, as if I don't have the engagement to listen to you.
- Yes, I feel left. Lonely.
  Anne thinks for a while. She realizes that another feeling has emerged.
- It's striking that right now I feel quite touched by your feeling of abandonment.

David and Anne have reached a point where the feeling of abandonment has taken shape between them. The position where they were stuck can be described as pretend mode. It could also be described as a teleological position, where telling childhood memories becomes a ritual for showing that therapy is going on.

By disclosing her feeling, Anne creates a new situation of abandoning and loneliness. Anne did not have any intention to create these feelings, she only felt uncertain about the meaningfulness of what they were doing. Other feelings could have come into focus, like anger or shame. By her openness, she made it possible to break the pretend mode between them and they started mentalizing around their relationship.

How to do in practice

In mentalizing-oriented therapies, mentalizing is often seen as a mental skill to be developed. However, mentalizing is also a stance towards life, characterized by curiosity, tolerance for uncertainty, and engagement in relationships. Contrasts to mentalizing are to be caught in enactments, to be excessively presumptuous, not to become emotionally involved.

In the illustration about David, pretend mode and teleological stance were illustrated. Psychic equivalence is often a more difficult situation to handle. In dyadic psychic equivalence, the participants become locked in their certainty. An illustration:

The patient is a young man who has been in therapy for a while because he feels depressed. At times he has suicidal thoughts, but he has never tried to act on them. He had a difficult upbringing with a drug abusing mother and an older brother who maltreated him regularly. Now he has a part time job as a janitor. He is certain that the maltreatment by his brother has made him feel inadequate in relationships. His therapist often has the impression that he is gawky with friends and girls.

- I met some friends yesterday and took some beers. But they joked about me most of the time, so I went home.
  The therapist thinks that she can see his awkwardness. She always tries to hearten him when this kind of situations come up.
- Isn't there someone among the who supports you? You might try to become more friendly with those who are kind to you.
- I do my best but there isn't really anyone.
  Again, the therapist gets an image of the patient as a shy and frightened boy. She feels resigned and tired. But she realizes that she has a quite limited picture of him. They seem to agree on not believing that he might stand up for himself. She decides to try a new perspective.
- I wonder what would happen if you just told them to stop.
- They would just laugh at me.
  The therapist senses a challenge.
- Are you certain? Did you try?
- Perhaps not all the way. But I know them.
- In some way, I think you have persuaded me about your vulnerability. I'd like to insist that you try.
- You make it too simple; you don't understand.

The session continues with the therapist provoking the patient to become more confident. When the patient hesitates, the disagreement between them becomes a possibility to explore conflictual feelings.

20 See the patient from the outside

The tool

It is a natural therapist reaction to see the patient's world from his per-spective, to empathize with him, sometimes also to validate his experience, to confirm the adequacy of his reactions. The exhortation to understand the patient from his perspective is strong, with support in Kierkegaard's motto: "In order truly to help someone else, I must understand more than he – but certainly first and foremost understand what he understands".

The other perspective, the complementary position, to see the patient from the outside, means two things: one is to pay attention to the reactions that the patient elicits in the therapist, the other is to be curious about how the patient describes how others react to him.

Complementary countertransference is not a blueprint of others' reac-tions to the patient. The tensions between how others react, and the therapist's reactions are important. The patient who describes that his father is constantly annoyed at him for asking for help may have a therapist who has noticed that the patient constantly wants advice but who likes to give them.

The purpose

The therapist may advise the patient with the prescription: "Put a limit on your boss's demands on you!" But how does she know that the manager's demands are unreasonable? The therapist may want to say: "You have to be clear to your partner that you want to talk with her". But the partner may in fact be quite eager to talk although the patient does not hear it. She might invite him to say: "Your children cannot know what is right for you". But the children may have important things to say. An important aspect of therapy is to help patient see himself through the eyes of others, to increase his sense for the meaningfulness of reflecting on others' views of him. One purpose is to understand others' reactions, another is to help him recognize the other's subjectivity.

DOI: 10.4324/9781003026914-20

The dilemma

The suggestion to talk rather spontaneously in relational therapy can be hazardous. The spontaneity may lead to unpremeditated support, unreflected sympathy for the patient. A reticent therapist stance can be a healthy stop bloc against automatic and unexamined validation of the patient's views.

As a remedy and protection to this risk, it may be helpful to hear what other persons think about the patient in order to get a perspective on one's own reactions. "His friends react with frustration to his self-centered and slightly narcissistic manners. Perhaps I have been trapped into considering him to be a cozy and nice boy". Or "I feel kind of warm feelings about his somewhat confusing way of talking but I hear that his friends get quite annoyed about him".

Differences in reactions may serve as important possibilities to detect nuances. "Someone is irritated about the patient's petulance. The therapist also feels irritated, but she also has a tenderness for the vulnerability she senses. She thinks about reasons for her tenderness. She realizes that her son also has a tendency to become kinky, but they have found ways to joke about it. She probably carries this forbearance over to the patient". A nuanced view of the countertransference may be helped by reports about others' reactions.

Principles

Empathy, interpreted as seeing the world from the patient's perspective, is a therapeutic, professional position. In everyday interaction, it is rather the person's own wishes, needs, in relation to the other, that are in focus. A person gets angry if the other does not fulfil her wishes, she may be sad when the other thwarts her longings. Therapeutic empathy is a professional approach, a step into a therapeutic stance, a mental repositioning. Consider the situation when two friends talk about everyday matters. Both of them bring their own ideas, use their own perspectives. When one of them says to the other that he has serious problems and wants to share them with his friend, the friend deliberately takes a new position, tries to see things from the other's perspective.

Derailed supportiveness?

A recurrent critique of relational therapy has been that the focus of the therapist is not on unconscious intentions and fantasies; it stays on the conscious, visible aspects of the patient's material. Relational therapy has been accused of being too supportive, to treat the patient as a victim of hardships and relational traumas. It encourages sympathy with the patient instead of analyzing his problems, replacing empathy with empathism (Bolognini, 1997).

It is probably true that an active therapist easily identifies with consciously experienced aspects of the patient. Traumatic experiences, negligence, and abandonment may easily evoke sympathetic feelings in the therapist and reflexive blaming of perpetrators. The therapist might, especially if she becomes engaged and upset, find it natural to stand on the patient's side.

This may be adequate. However, the background of hardships may be more complicated than the patient's formulations suggest, both patient and therapist may be blind about the patient's agency in traumatic situations, the consequences in the patient's mind may be more shameful than he may be able to tell. The patient often has a more complicated perspective of what happened than the therapist. An important dilemma in work with trauma survivors is to strike a balance between validation of the victim's experiences and exploration of the patient's experience of his subjectivity.

In emotionally and ethically complicated sorting out of memories and feelings of traumatic situations, the forgiving aspect of relational therapy is that enacted reactions are also material. Excessive sympathy and empathism are interactional problems that can be used for reflection.

The allure in recognizing patterns

To search for reaction patterns is natural and often fruitful. But scouting for similarities should be tempered by openness to be surprised by the ongoing interaction, pattern seeking mitigated by eagerness to be astonished. "He is a kind man, but he is unbearably long-winded. I can't stop being irritated although I know that he has a good heart. His wife apparently found his circumstantiality enervating as she left him". This is fine as a guess, an assumption. If it becomes certainty, it is psychic equivalence. Psychotherapy is not a jigsaw puzzle or a detective challenge, pieces should not fit together. The challenge is not to fill the slots in Malan's triangle. All too often, therapy becomes intellectual, the patient may feel unmasked, the case is solved. If others have reacted in the same way as the therapist, it is thought-provoking. But it is not a solution.

David

David's uncle and aunt have three children. Most of the time in childhood, David liked them and played with them. But during several years, the oldest of the cousins, a boy four years older than David, subjected him to various harassments. He teased him, hit him, and on some occasions, he molested David sexually. David felt that he made it to show his power, to humiliate him. He had not thought much about it later, and now they had a bearable relationship.

When the therapist challenged David about his feelings towards his colleague Inga's demonstrations of her knowledge, the question of previous humiliations came up and, after some probing, she realized the extent of the

cousin's abuse. David had talked with his mother about the verbal harassments when they occurred. As he felt that she minimized what he said, he
never talked about the sexual abuse. When Anne asked about them, David
was avoidant. After some probing, David talked about how his cousin had
taken him to a forest in the neighborhood and forced him to fellatio. Anne
realized that this had indeed been traumatic for him. David was not very
happy talking about it. After Anne had insisted, he recalled that the cousin
had said derogatory things about him. David especially remembered that he
had said things about his mother and the men she met, and about his father.
In David's world, there was no one to turn to for help.

–   What did you say to your mother?
–   I think I said something about him saying nasty things to me. She
    wasn't very interested, she said that some boys do that.
–   So you didn't try again?
–   I tried a few times. But I thought it might be difficult for her if I couldn't
    be at my uncle's place.
–   So you thought you had to stand it for her sake?
–   Well, I thought it would be hard for her to know that they were not kind
    to me.
    *Anne tries to catch her reflections. She has the same feeling as when he
    talks about his colleague: he is hesitant to tell the whole story.*
–   You must have felt lonely at that time. No one knew about it.
–   I guess it was ok that I kept it to myself.
–   Do you want me to know about this? It struck me that it is me who
    takes the initiative. It becomes kind of an interview.
–   It's no fun to talk about it. And I wonder what you think of me? I guess
    you might look down on me.
    *Does Anne think that David should stand up for himself in relation to
    Inga? Yes, she does. It may also be that his mother thought he should have
    stopped the cousin. Is there a common theme in David's way of recounting
    his degrading experiences? Anne wonders if his mother may have asked
    more than he wants to remember, that she may have felt dismissed.*

As the dialogue continues, Anne tries to ask David about his fantasies of her
thoughts about his hesitance to talk and makes some disclosures about her
own feelings. During the following sessions, they talk about what happened
with the cousin but primarily about David's unwillingness to confide in
anyone, and about feelings of shame for getting humiliated. The conversation shows similarities as well as differences between the situations.

How to do in practice?

In many therapies, the relational implications of the patient's problems are
obvious. A person who loses his temper may be hard to live with, and at

occasions also to have as a patient. But with other kinds of problems, the therapist may have to make an effort in her fantasy in order to understand the relational consequences.

Anxiety is an example. Variants of anxiety disorders are often seen as the individual's own problem, reactions to be unconditioned, behaviour to be relearned. Standard treatments focus on exposure and behaviour experiments, exercises that the individual patient can make on his own.

Using a relational perspective, it is apparent that it often may be difficult to live with persons with anxiety problems. A partner standing in the shower an hour to make sure all soap is washed away or getting out of bed several times every evening to make sure the door is really locked is certainly provocative. The common CBT treatment for obsessions, response prevention, is a systematization of the understandable folk psychology admonition: "Stop your self-defeating behavior!"

An illustration

- I was really trying to do as you said. I had decided to take just a short shower. But in the end, I stood there for more than half an hour.
- What did your girlfriend say?
- She says she feels sorry for me. But I guess she is irritated. I hope she understands me. I try to do my best.
  The patient has tried to limit his compulsive behaviour a number of times. The therapist by now is pretty fed up but also feels sorry for the patient.
- It's pretty similar for me. You know, I do think that you try. But I think it is important to understand what happens with people around you. Looking from your inside, you struggle to limit your behaviour. Looked at from the outside, people like your girlfriend and I might think: "Just stop it, what's the problem".
- So you think it's an easy thing for me?

The spontaneous conversation has landed in a suggestion of anger and disappointment in the patient. To some extent, the therapist has provoked it by expressing a natural reaction to the patient's behaviour. The therapist does not probe the girlfriend's reaction in order to show that frustration or irritation should be the only possible reactions but to focus on them in order to help the patient start thinking that his behaviour does have relational consequences. The purpose is to open for curiosity about relational meanings of a rigid behaviour. It is not to find unconscious reasons for the behaviour, for example, anger directed towards others concealed as compulsive anxiety.

Possibilities of the complementary position

When the therapist tries to understand the patient, it may go from the simple: "My sympathy for her may be an indication that she averts conflicts" or "Does she want me to be irritated because she is afraid I might like her?" to more sophisticated guesses: "My cautiousness might suggest that we have created an image that she is vulnerable in order not to approach a genuine contact that we may find temptatious". When such reactions become formulated to the patient, they may evoke quite different forms of dyadic engagement. They may lead to enactments, but it may also open for potential space exploration (Benjamin, 1990, 2017).

Sometimes, comparisons with others' reactions may make it easier for the patient to understand the reason for the therapist's disclosures of her reactions. "I heard you saying that your girlfriend sometimes finds your face tense. My reaction is perhaps somewhat similar, but I think I sense a sensitivity in your face".

A useful way to use others' perspective as food for reflection is for the therapist to consider what she would feel if she met the patient a lot more than she does. The observation "He is bumptious but not more than I can stand it. However, if he were my partner or child, I would get extremely irritated" is a good start for explorations of the interaction.

21 See yourself from within

The tool

In order to help a patient, the therapist has to find a place in herself where she can recognize the patient's struggle. Understanding the patient requires that the therapist makes available an intersubjective space that the patient may use, a space where the therapist can find something in herself that is similar enough to the patient's suffering. When the therapist tries to catch the reactions evoked by the patient, she will soon realize that her reactions are not just reactions to the patient, they have roots in her own experiences, they are images from her life, reflections of her own relational sensitivities, feelings that she is accustomed to feel. The therapist understands the patient by finding him in her own life. If the patient changes, the therapist also changes to some extent.

The purpose

Relational therapy is not about teaching a technique to reach a goal. It is about striving to enlarge the patient's understanding of his emotional and relational situation. If the therapist wants to help a patient with his life problems, they must become problems for her as well. Not always in the same way as for the patient. Not always only in a friendly or empathic way. She may experience him as annoying or querulous or seductive or boring. But she has to let him take hold of her mentally, get into her (or experience the resistance to letting him in). Unless some aspect of the patient's suffering becomes alive and meaningful to the therapist, connects to her own life struggles in some way, there will be no relational treatment.

The dilemma

The focus of therapy is the patient. The patient's problems are the reason for the contact. What if the understanding of the patient's problems must be coloured by the therapist's understanding? What if the therapist makes the

DOI: 10.4324/9781003026914-21

patient struggle with her own problem? What if issues of separation, or death, or shame, are of the therapist's?

The therapist's recognition of the patient's problems takes place from her perspective. Although most therapists have felt unjustified fear, hopelessness, anxiety about being left, most of them have not lost a child or been psychotic. But we can understand how it might feel. The desperation in a parent who loses his child cannot be known to anyone who has not had that experience, but we may try to imagine what it would be like.

The Swedish poet Gunnar Ekelöf wrote: "What is the bottom in you is the bottom also of others" in the poem *The Lonely Man*. Existentially, the common bottom is life's conditions, for each person with its own forms and expressions. To long for closeness, to feel abandoned, to find meaning in life, to be aware of one's vulnerability.

But from another perspective, the therapist does not and cannot identify with the patient's problem. The patient's distinctiveness rather becomes a problem. He may create situations where she feels caught, pressured, and enamored. Sometimes, this is the kind of experience that is called projective identification in one-person object relations theory. Sometimes, it is less constrained. But she is different from the patient, separate. It shows the essential uniqueness of every person that Levinas describes.

Principles

"With every therapeutic encounter, therapists must courageously confront themselves and expand their awareness of themselves in relation to yet another individual. The therapeutic process should, therefore, involve change for both participants" (Muran, 2007, p. 262).

This citation points to the personal challenge that each relational therapy implies. To describe humans' unavoidable fate, Heidegger (1927) used the phrase "Geworfenheit", to be thrown into the world. This also pertains to genuine psychotherapy. We cannot stand outside; we cannot only observe. To be a *participating* observer (Sullivan, 1940) is not only advice; it is a necessity. Participation is to get immersed, thrown into it. If meta-communication is to comment on the interaction from the outside, in some objective sense, it is always only failed attempts. All understanding is based on idiosyncratic images, creating new interactional complexities (Ogden, 1994a).

Personal therapy may improve the therapist's sensitivity and awareness of painful aspects of relationships, partly replace fear and bewilderment with curiosity. The repertoire of tolerable memories may become wider. But they are still personal to the therapist, she has no other life than her own. In serious emotional commitments, we are at the mercy of the brick stones that our life has given us. The therapist's influence on the therapeutic material cannot be parceled out or seen as bias. The patient's narratives are co-created with the therapist. From the therapist's perspective, "it is one's own understanding, based on one's own assumptions about human life, one's own dynamics" (Mitchell, 1998, p. 20). According to Bollas (1987), each patient brings his own "personal idiom" to the therapy. So does the therapist.

The therapist's vulnerability

The patient comes to therapy with his vulnerability. It is not always apparent on the outside, but no patient comes to serious therapy without open or unacknowledged vulnerability. To help him, his therapist must find vulnerability in herself that is close enough to the patient's (DiAmbrosio, 2014; Mitchell, 1998; Silverman, 2019; Sirote, 2020). This is particularly evident in work with psychotic patients (Ogden, 1989; Searles, 1975) and with patients with severe trauma. Searles (1975) argued that severely disturbed patients need to experience that their observation of the therapist's emotional fragility is confirmed and accepted by her. Sometimes, the patient's disavowed mental struggles are first visible in the therapist's experience together with the patient (Ogden, 1989).

David

David has visited his mother during the weekend. She has recently retired. Although she has some old friends, she lives a lonely life. David often has guilt feelings about not visiting more often. However, he detests to just sit there talking with her, he cannot figure out what to talk about and he has heard a thousand times what she has to say. This time she told him that she had met David's uncle. The uncle is eager to help David's mother. Sometimes he invites her to various events. Now he was going to a clothes outlet and wanted her to join. But she does not want, she has no money, she does not need any new clothes, and she feels humiliated by his invitation.

- She seems to get stuck in her loneliness and feelings of abandonment.
- It's no wonder she doesn't go along. Why should she? My uncle can get really debasing when he says he wants to take care of her.
- You're still very occupied by your feelings about him. I thought it was quite some time since he was patronizing towards her. I realize it was tough, but she, and you, might find new ways of being with him.
- You think so? You think she can leave that behind?
  David sounds irritated. Anne thinks about how to continue. The idea that David's mother should get over her humiliation was no good. David is strongly identified with his mother in this. Anne thinks it is a destructive grievance.
- You don't get tired of this feeling of humiliation?
- You mean I should just forget it?
- Or rather accept it as something that happened a long time ago.
  David is silent. Anne thinks it would be good to insist.

- Of course, it was hard for you. But you can't let all your life be dominated by these feelings of degradation.
  David is again silent for some seconds.
- You don't seem to understand. I don't think you've been in such a situation.
- Perhaps not, although I've had my share. But your mother's feelings are one thing. What about you? Could you let it be?
- It is as if you want me to ignore her feelings, just tell her to skip them.
- You mean you have an obligation to listen to your mother's disappointments?
- It goes under my skin. I've felt sad since I saw her.
- I thought you sounded angry when you described your feelings when you meet her.
  David is silent. Anne's thoughts turn to her own mother. Her mother had a high position in a company but was sacked for alleged duty neglect when Anne was in her teens. She often ruminates about her grievances. For several years, Anne has thought that she has had enough of it. She identified with her mother when it happened, but since a long time she feels she has left it.

They continue talking about David's feelings. Anne becomes aware that she does not really get hold of what David is struggling with. Her own mother often tells her that she is insensitive and hard when the mother talks about her life. After the session, Anne realizes that she may have become stuck in a kind of stubbornness towards her.

How to do in practice?

The therapist's imaginative resources

When you read a novel, environments and people emerge and become alive. Where do the images come from? From your own life. When you listen to a patient describing his partner, his children, his separation, the images created in your mind come from your own life. We cannot create images of what we do not see with our own eyes unless we use the memories and fantasies that are in us.

This is an automatic process. It is obvious that Anne's own life experiences colour her understanding of David's situation. Traditionally, the therapist's feelings have been put aside as the therapist's countertransference, or used as food for thought as possible indications of projective identification (Ogden, 1994b). The spontaneity in relational therapy invites to a more vital dialogue, but the colouring of the dialogue by the therapist's own images also opens for hurdles, as shown in the illustration with David.

The therapist's change

A leading idea in relational therapy is that change takes place intersubjectively. "Both client and therapist are mutually but asymmetrically shaped and transformed over time as a function of their responsibilities and roles" (Atzil-Slonim & Tschacher, 2020, p. 555). This idea is not normative, it is not an exhortation. It is a lived experience in therapists and a consequence of the therapeutic model. It would indeed be presumptuous to require that the therapist should change.

The therapist's loneliness – an illustration

The patient's presented problem at the primary care service is panic attacks. After some unsuccessful attempts with education and exposure, the patient starts talking about his marriage. Some years ago, his wife had a life-threatening tumour. She is medically cured but under strict control as relapses are usual with this cancer type. The therapist herself had a similar tumour a few years back. She knows about the risks; she knows the percentage of five-year survival. She is mentally prepared, and scared, for the potential relapse. Without disclosing anything about her own medical state, she is full of feelings when her patient talks about his worries.

The therapist also has a partner; she has thought a lot about what will happen with him if she dies. Recently, the thought overwhelmed her that her partner would find a new partner. She felt unreasonably jealous at the thought. She tried to figure out whom he might become interested in. She tried to control herself and spoke with him. He became angry and disappointed and assured her that he was only focused on her, other thoughts were simply not imaginable to him. She felt stupid and regretted that she had suggested anything of the kind. But she retained the fantasies.

At their last session, the therapist was quite occupied with ideas about the attractiveness of her patient. She thinks he looks young and vigorous, and she listens attentively about anything that suggests that he might be interested in other women. When he talks about a conversation with a colleague, the therapist gets the impression that he might have liked her, she hints at potential romantic feelings. He follows suit, confirms that he likes her. They talk about his relationship with her and other women.

At the next session, he is angry. He has realized that the therapist suggested that he might want to have an erotic relationship with the other woman. He wants to firmly declare that he has no such thoughts. The therapist feels ashamed. She realizes that she has had the same kind of thoughts about her patient as about her husband. She does not say anything to the patient about this link but admits that she may have influenced him in a way that was not important to him, that her fantasies may have led her astray.

During the following sessions, the talk moves around the patient's feelings about his wife. He reflects on the impossibility to fully understand how it feels to have a potentially fatal illness.

Engaged therapy is created by the needs and fears of the participants. In this example, the therapist was unusually occupied by an issue that also became relevant to the patient, but with other key signatures. Openly or surreptitiously, they engage in issues that are important to them. Although problematic, the dialogue gets energy from the importance of the issue for the therapist. Sometimes, the therapist's own engagement may be felt to be too strong; it is a challenge to know when disclosure might be to the benefit of the patient.

22 How to develop as a relational psychotherapist

Relational therapy has two overarching goals: development of the patient's relational skills and increased ability to lead a more vital, meaningful, and authentic life. Although obviously simplified, this distinction also points to different ways for therapists to improve their professional competence. This is not to say that therapist training has to follow two distinct tracks. But for heuristic purposes, it is helpful to discuss therapist development using these perspectives.

Although *relational skills* are rooted in the personality, have a constitutional base, and have developed during a long life, it is possible to develop such skills. Trying to be sensitive to and aware of one's own and others' feelings, finding new and more nuanced words for them are skills that can be practised in different relational contexts. To be mindful in relationships, to attend to problems in them, and to reflect on what it would imply to communicate about them is possible to train.

Authenticity and *genuineness* are not skills; neither is *emotional presence*. They are fundamental approaches to oneself and one's fellow humans. Approaches to life cannot be exercised. Personal therapy, supervision, reflections on decisive and profound life experiences are ways to develop as a person. For many, being a therapist is an important way to develop as a person (Råbu & McLeod, 2018). Experiences of therapeutic encounters may be highly vitalizing and of significance for the rest of life. But we do not consider them as training opportunities. They enrich our lives.

The concept training in this context has an ethical significance. Suppose that I offer a more delicious meal than usually to my family. No one is offended if I tell them that I have found a good cooking course online. But if I become more loving than usually towards my loved one and tell her that I have taken an online course in love, she would not be happy. We have with reason ambivalent feelings for exercises about relationship skills and abilities like closeness, authenticity, presence, intimacy, and love. It may be understandable that there are courses in how to make friends, how to engage with angry children. But a course in intimacy? In authenticity?

DOI: 10.4324/9781003026914-22

Accountability

A therapist has legal duty and moral responsibility not to disseminate information about what the patient tells her. A patient has good reason to assume that what he talks about is a secret between him and his therapist. The patient should be able to tell the therapist what he cannot tell his partner. "Sometimes I look at violent and humiliating pornography", "Sometimes I get scared about impulses to hurt children", "Sometimes thoughts just pop up in my head and I feel that they are not mine". It is reasonable that the patient wants the therapist to keep such information to herself. The same goes for peek experiences in the therapy relationship. As with other intimate and confidential experiences, they should stay with the therapeutic couple.

This is one perspective. The other is that most people seek help because they want to get rid of symptoms or problems or because they want to feel less restricted in some respect. Most patients are not experts on how psychotherapy should be conducted and often cannot judge whether the therapist delivers it in a competent way. In medical treatment, it is natural that more than one person has insight into the treatment and that the treatment is followed up in a way that can be evaluated objectively. Even if the problem should be embarrassing or complicated, patients want the best help.

We have confidential talks with our friends or with priests. But psychotherapy is not friendship or confession, it is a paid service. Some authors argue that if the therapist is well trained, the patient can trust that the treatment is good enough. Others contend that supervision is a guarantee for correct treatment. These are not good arguments. There are plenty of examples, including well-known therapists and published studies, of failed and poorly managed treatments (Wise & Barnett, 2016). The therapist chooses what to present to the supervisor; supervisory relationships not seldom become colluded.

The conflict between the patient's right to a confidential therapy relationship and his right to know that the treatment is professional enough is a real dilemma. It is, of course, possible to talk with the patient about it, but that is with the knowledge that the patient is in a dependent position and may refrain from expressing questions and doubts. The demands for accountability in the psychotherapy world are increasing, for good reasons.

The therapist factor

Therapists differ substantially in their average outcome results (Johns, Barkham, Kellett, & Saxon, 2019; Saxon, Firth, & Barkham, 2016; Wampold & Imel, 2015). This therapist effect seems to be larger with more severely disturbed patients (Saxon & Barkham, 2012) and in therapies with more sessions. Already at fifteen sessions, high-performing therapists are twice as effective as low-performing. Patients of high-performing therapists continue to improve at each session, whereas the improvement of patients of low-performing therapists stagnate (Goldberg, Hoyt, Nissen-Lie, Nielsen, & Wampold, 2018). Although patient characteristics influence the alliance, a significant share of outcome variance seems to be due to differences in therapists' ability to create a viable alliance (Del Re, Flückiger, Horvath, & Wampold, 2021).

Relational skills rather than technical ability probably contribute to outcome variation among therapists (Laska et al., 2014; Wampold & Owen, in press). In this area, we are at a crossroads of sorts between official requirements and research findings. While authorities and training providers emphasize that adherence to technique is crucial, research convincingly demonstrates that a large proportion of treatment results depend on the individual therapist's ability to establish a constructive and creative treatment relationship with the individual patient, and that therapists differ in this regard, independent of treatment method.

Empirical studies do not show that longer experience and more formal training enhance therapists' results (Goldberg et al., 2016). Patients of less experienced therapists seem, in fact, to improve marginally more than patients of more experienced therapists. Although such findings may be open to sceptical objections about difficulties to measure, it is unquestionably troublesome that there is no systematic evidence for the advantage of experience or training.

Perhaps therapists should be selected on their relational skills before they are accepted for professional training, as are musicians or artists? In this, there is a complicated paradox. Although available research indicates that inherent ability, probably based on genetic disposition and acquired personality, is the primary foundation for relational skills, we consider competencies like enhanced mentalizing and larger availability of affects to be central goals of therapy. It would indeed be strange if we as therapists try to help our patients develop such capacities but do not believe that therapists may change.

One reason for the lack of therapist experience advantage in outcome studies could be that newer therapists have stronger curiosity about and engagement in the individual patient. Professional stagnation seems to be a common problem among therapists who have worked many years (Rønnestad & Skovholt, 2013).

Expertise and experience

During its history, psychotherapy has been preoccupied by the issue of therapy method versus therapist. Kiesler (1966) cautioned about attempts to see therapists and the therapy process as uniform. However, the idea that therapists may, like engineers, identify recurring processes in the patient's material and apply techniques to change them has a long history in both CBT and psychodynamic therapies (McWilliams, 1999, 2004; OPD, 2008; Summers & Barber, 2014). In the CCRT tradition, for instance, the idea is that recurrent interpersonal patterns are possible to identify (Crits-Christoph, Barber, & Kurcias, 1993) in a reliable way by any good therapist. Likewise, the idea in Safran's and Muran's (2000) model for rupture resolutions is that ruptures basically reflect the patient's maladaptive interpersonal patterns. Resolution of ruptures contribute to more constructive ways to handle them in other relationships. Although the therapist is supposed to show humility and to admit contributions to ruptures, it is still a technical competence, possible to improve.

The empirical findings that therapists do not improve their results over time make the idea that technical competence is the crux for effective therapy less probable. Technical skills, meaning interventions that evoke a detectable response or a reaction within a reasonable time limit, may improve, but not to the long-term benefit of the patient. A reason may be that the effects that therapy is supposed to lead grow slowly and, to a large extent, unpredictably. The recipe for developing expertise in the sense of skills competence is a world with regular patterns, many opportunities to train a specific behaviour, and immediate feedback. (Kahneman, 2011; Shanteau, 1992).

None of these factors is common in psychotherapy. Each situation is new, feedback in any useful sense is opaque. The possibility to distinguish long-term effects of manual-guided technical interventions from the effects of tailor-made approaches is small.

In such situations, there is an apparent risk that the therapist's own ideas of specific therapeutic stances inflate their belief in their method and lead to confirmation bias. Ideas of therapist expertise and proficiency becomes an ideological rather than an empirical question. It is thoughtworthy that therapists with more professional self-doubt attain better results than those who are cocksure about their ability (Nissen-Lie et al., 2017).

Relational qualities in therapists

Despite the uncertainty about what constitutes therapist expertise, some relational abilities seem significant for effective therapy. Are they possible to improve? From the minute response in an interaction to the successive building of a confidential relationship, relational skills are among the most difficult challenges for humans. Binder and Strupp (1997) commented on the "enormous difficulty that human beings, even highly trained therapists, have in dealing with interpersonal conflict in which they are participants" (p. 123). And not only to deal with conflicts. All skills needed to handle complicated relational situations are hard to train. Anderson and colleagues (2016a, 2016b) found that facilitative interpersonal skills such as verbal fluency, emotional expressiveness, persuasiveness, hopefulness, warmth, empathy, bond-creating capacity, and problem focus, rated on trainees' responses to simulated therapy vignettes before their therapy training started, predicted outcome after training. Unfortunately, training did not improve the skills.

Mentalizing

Mentalizing has been suggested as a key competence for therapists. Probably, mentalizing in the interaction between patient and therapist is an important condition for change in many therapy methods. Although, as noted in Chapter 19, mentalizing may best be seen as an interactional phenomenon, the therapist's ability to mentalize may have importance. In a study of therapists' mentalizing ability, Cologon, Schweitzer, King, and Nolte (2017) found that 70% of the variation between therapists with regard to average symptom improvement in their patients could be accounted for by differences in their mentalizing capacity.

The main issue is probably the quality of mentalizing in the particular dialog. Diamond, Stovall-McClough, Clarkin, and Levy (2003), in a study of transference-focused therapy, found that best results were attained when therapists were one step ahead of the patient, but not more, in explicit reflective functioning. Several studies have found that a therapist's reflective functioning in relation to a particular patient is associated with her ability to identify and resolve alliance ruptures (Reading, Safran, Origlieri, & Muran, 2019). Interestingly, patients of therapists with better mentalizing ability did not achieve better outcome at treatment termination; neither did the patients report better alliance. However, at follow up, more reflective therapists had better outcome. A reason could be that therapists who are better at mentalizing tend to be more challenging as they discover more subtle ruptures in the therapeutic cooperation. The effects of mentalizing rupture restorations seem to come with some latency.

Genuineness

Exercises in how to become more genuine in human contacts, more authentic in affective expressions may sound like a contradictio in adiecto, an attempt to fake humanness. The issue is a real dilemma. No one would like to have a lover who had been trained in lover's qualities. On the other hand, psychotherapy would be an odd profession if the main qualification, to be a genuine person, is a quality that cannot be developed. Questioning whether the spontaneity and authenticity necessary for psychotherapeutic change can be taught, Stern (2004b) wrote: "Yes and no. Once the general idea about change processes ... has been taught and assimilated, one gains a different perspective or vision about the process one is engaged in. It is this shift in perspective that makes the difference". (p. 372). However, authenticity may more often be professed than effectively practised (Stern, 2015, p. 392). Consider the difficulty in evaluating one's own degree of authenticity!

Tolerance for uncertainty

Psychoanalysis has made a great leap during hundred years from the idea that there are correct interpretations of repressed intentions to the contemporary stance of not knowing, of emphasis on the therapist's epistemological openness, in a somewhat paradoxical contrast to several other psychotherapy methods whose representatives used to criticize psychoanalysis for rigid adherence to improbable interpretations. Even systematic theories are seen as possibilities to use, tools that may be tried and replaced (Mitchell, 1997). The tool is not The Theory, but the engagement in the committed search for meaning and value together with the patient, using theories in a pragmatic way.

There are many ways of not knowing. Socratic questioning implies a position of asking questions instead of presenting answers. In therapy, it means to stimulate the patient to cultivate a scientific stance towards himself. In relational therapy, the basic stance is mutual and engaged curiosity on what goes on in the interaction. "Knowing what to do may be very important, doing this with certainty is not in itself a realistic ambition, and being able to not know what to do may well be the most crucial skill" (Seligman, 2014, p. 653).

Genuine curiosity is not only about the patient, but also about the therapist's own, often unwitting, participation. The therapist "hopes to create thoughtful and emotionally responsive understandings of the patient herself, and the ongoing clinical process; but she also hopes to maintain a radical uncertainty that, when necessary, will allow her to reimagine these understandings as unconscious participations with the patient" (Stern, 2015, p. 390). Attempts to understand are natural in therapy. Not so natural are attempts to deconstruct understanding, regarding it as dyadic defenses against uncertainty.

David

For a time, Anne had felt that she was not affected by David's struggles to find a way back to life in the way that she expected. She felt numb even as he talked about experiences that seemed sad or could have upset her. When David recounted how his cousins had teased him because he had no father, Anne realized that he must have felt quite lonely. Scenes were created before her eyes, but she did not become touched, she felt rather bored.

She had talked with David about her reactions. They found that Anne's reactions were similar to those he had felt from his mother. They reflected on Anne's and potentially the mother's guilt feelings about not being moved and David's anger and sense of hopelessness.

The dialogue was fruitful. David had shown his anger and disappointment, Anne had formulated thoughts about David becoming a victim. But afterwards, Anne had felt the conversation to be stylized, predictable. She decided to talk with someone else about her reaction. She took it up with her supervisor. Together, they reflected on whether Anne's life situation could give some clues. They compared with the supervision relationship. The supervisor became aware of his own subtle sense of irritation about Anne's overly ambitious attempts to be sensitive at all times. "Calm down!" the supervisor wanted to say. "You can't be empathic always". They talked about this side of Anne's professional self. Anne thought about ambitiousness in her life. She knew that one reason of her choice profession was the wish to be helpful to people, to show warmth and interest in a sometimes exaggerated way, with roots in her life.

Anne pondered about this for some days. She talked with a friend who admitted that at times she felt Anne's well-meaning questions to be intrusive. She could sometimes feel that Anne was too eager to be emotionally responsive, that it was Anne's needs rather than the friend's situation that was in focus. One evening, Anne and her partner started by chance to look at a film about homeless children in Venezuela. She realized that this was the kind of situation where she might feel sympathetic in a somewhat egocentric way. She agreed with her partner that they would stop the film at intervals and talk about their feelings. Although her partner liked her empathic approach very much, he also commented that he did not find her sympathy quite genuine at times.

At the next supervision session, her supervisor suggested that Anne might select a few psychotherapy sessions from expert therapists on the internet, look at them and try to imagine what the patients might feel. When Anne came back, she reported that she had felt rather irritated by the intrusiveness exhibited by some of the therapists. But there were others who she felt were truly considerate about their patients.

When Anne met David the next time, David talked about grievances he had felt at his workplace. Anne was observant about her potential tendency to become sympathetic. Or blasé. She asked for details in order to try to catch her feelings. The dialogue became nuanced; Anne found that she had regained her feeling repertoire, she could feel more than sympathy or detachment.

Training

Foucault argued that techniques are only partly transferable by communication or attainable by training or education (Martin, Gutman, & Hutton, 1988). Psychodynamic training traditionally consists of theoretical discussions, personal therapy, and supervision. Psychoanalytic "stances" like Freud's admonition of "freely floating attention" (Freud, 1912) and Bion's dictum "to listen without memory and desire" (Bion, 1970) are guidelines for the psychoanalytic therapist's mindset. Current understanding of intersubjective processes has pointed to the complicated and basically unrealistic nature of such ideals (Davies, 2018). There is no therapist without memory and desire (Slavin & Kriegman, 1998); the therapist always contributes to the co-creation of the mutual understanding.

Another aspect of psychoanalytic training has for a long time decided its direction: the school. Ever since psychoanalytic therapists began to identify with different theoretical camps, it has been important to provide the beginning therapist with the correct model of the mind. Kleinian therapists have been taught to interpret the patient's material along the line of early phantasies; Kohutians are trained to understand how the therapist serves as a self-object and to show appropriate empathy in order for the patient to develop his mature narcissism. Psychoanalytic training has during its existence emphasized "correct" ways of using techniques. There has been an obvious lack of curiosity on other ways of working, arguably starting in the disputes and exclusions in the small Viennese psychoanalytic group.

Belief in such restricted models of the mind seems outdated. Slavin (2007b) calls for an observer perspective, a "third" view on technique. Psychological models are possibilities, not truths (Mitchell, 1997). Instead of looking for the "correct" way of understanding the patient's problem, the therapist may have a storehouse of options that can be negotiated with the patient (Aron, 2018). At one time, the patient may need a rational advice, or a practical tool, at another, an idea of the childhood background for the current problem. Attachment models may be tried; if they do not give meaning to the patient's predicaments, the oedipal conflict model may be of use. The therapist invites the patient to ideas that the therapist has at hand and that emerge in their interaction (Mitchell, 1997).

Another aspect of the therapist's freedom is to leave instructions behind. Reik (1949) compared the therapist with an actor: "The actor should, when he walks out upon the stage, forget what he has studied at the academy. He must brush it aside as if it had never been there. If he cannot neglect it now, in the moment of real performance – if it has not gone deep enough that he can afford to neglect it – then his training wasn't good enough" (p. 20). This may be true. But the challenge is the academy, the training leading up to expert performance.

Practice suggestions

Successful violinists train the same movement with the bow ten thousand times (Ericsson 2009). It has been suggested that abilities like being able to tolerate affects together with a patient or approaching traumatic narratives could be exercised in the same way. An important movement among contemporary psychotherapists is the idea of *deliberate practice* (Bennett-Levy, 2019; Rousmaniere, 2016) meaning that therapist reactions to complicated situations should be exercised repeatedly, both for skills training and for exposure to anxiety-provoking feelings. At least one empirical study corroborates this idea. Chow et al. (2015) found that time spent on focusing on patients, irrespective of activity, was associated with better patient outcome.

Training to become a better relational therapist focuses on two qualities and one overarching approach. The qualities are the ability to become emotionally engaged, moved, to have access to and tolerate a range of intense feelings, to immediacy, and the ability to reflect, to take a step back, to become curious. These qualities should be used within a mental context of non-dogmatism. The ideological identity should be narrow, the tolerance for uncertainty and joy of discovery large.

Mindfulness

An important therapeutic skill is presence in the relationship (Geller & Greenberg, 2012). Mindfulness training may improve the ability to be present (Crane et al., 2017; MacDonald & Muran, 2020). Grepmair et al. (2007) found that patients who were seen by their therapists immediately after the therapists' mindfulness meditation had better outcome than patients seen at other times.

Although mindfulness as a preparation for sessions may be constructive, the real challenge is to be mindful in the therapeutic interaction, to be mindful-in-action (Safran & Muran, 2000). There are no studies on the direct effects of therapist mindfulness meditation on the quality of the therapeutic relationship, but research does suggest that it may lead to less stress and burnout in therapists (Erikson, Germundsjö, Åström, & Rönnlund, 2018).

Some studies point to the usefulness of mindfulness meditation as session introduction for patients (Mander et al., 2019). It may probably be useful to do this meditation together with the therapist. In general, however, the impact of mindfulness mediation on therapists' mental health has been too little systematically studied (Lomas et al., 2018).

Self-compassion

Self-compassion therapies (Germer & Neff, 2019; Gilbert, 2005) emphasize the need to take care of oneself and to be self-soothing in times of perceived failure, inadequacy, and suffering, to treat oneself with warmth, to accept failures and shortcomings, to reframe critical self-talk, and to physically take care of oneself. The effects of self-compassion for therapists are still not studied to any great extent (Patsiopoulos & Buchanan, 2011).

Therapy monitoring systems

A car mechanic or a carpenter gets direct feedback from the accomplished task or from the customer. In psychotherapy, it is much more complicated to understand when the work does not move in the right direction. The therapy situation does not provide the therapist with much objective feedback, and it may be hard to evaluate the mutual work in a fair way. Therapists seem to avoid realizing that their patients' problems sometimes get worse (Hannan et al., 2005; Hatfield, McCullough, Frantz, & Krieger, 2010) and to overestimate their own competence. Walfish, McAlister, O'Donnell, and Lambert (2012) found that 25% of therapists considered themselves to be over the 90th percentile among therapists in competence. None considered herself to be below the mean.

As a way to improve therapists' ability to detect negative developments in therapy, systematic feedback systems have been developed during some decades. Such systems rely on patients' self-ratings of their symptoms and problems. The ratings are usually processed digitally and offered to the therapist as a graph of how the patient perceives his symptom and problems and, sometimes, what he thinks about the alliance.

The empirical results about the usefulness of feedback systems are equivocal. Recent research reviews indicate moderate to marginal effects (Delgadillo et al., 2018; Lambert, Whipple, & Kleinstäuber, 2018; Østergård, Randa, & Hougaard, 2020). Studies suggest that the systems have better effect when the therapists are dedicated to use them (de Jong, van Sluis, Nugter, Heiser, & Spinhoven, 2012) and when the patient is invited to share the graphs (Amble, Gude, Stubdal, Andersen, & Wampold, 2015).

Different reasons have been advanced for the lack of persuasive effects. Therapists may be unfamiliar with the use of the systems, reluctant to use them, or may consider the feedback information to lack precision or utility.

Using routine outcome monitoring (ROM), the patient usually rates his symptoms before each session and his perception of the alliance at the end of the session. Let us consider a patient who reports decrease of symptoms and stable alliance in the first sessions. The anxiety symptoms go down and he feels he can cope better with his difficulties. The patient and the therapist look together at the curves and are pleased with the development. After some more sessions, the curve does not turn downwards any longer. Instead, it even goes up a little bit. The therapist would reflect on the situation, perhaps together with the patient, and perhaps suggest some action to try to reverse the development. There may be aspects of the patient's problem they have missed, there may be something in the collaboration that does not fit. They might talk about the patient's motivation, evaluate his capacity for doing the therapeutic tasks, and consider other directions for the work.

With a relational perspective, the therapist would invite the patient to a joint reflection on what the ratings might mean and how they affect the interaction. The therapist may feel worried, she may wonder what the patient wants her to know, she may feel ashamed that she has not been able to help him. Alternatively, she may be content that the patient perceives the severity of his problems, that he is truer to himself. The ratings become material for shared reflection; the graphs are used as a mental playground, a dyadic potential space.

Filming sessions

It has become common to record sessions for supervision during training. Looking at filmed sessions may be important in order to become aware of mentalizing deficiencies, lacunae in affect awareness, and problematic ways of handling subtle alliance problems (Muran & Eubanks, 2020). Chow et al. (2015) found that it was particularly valuable if the therapist looked at video-recorded therapy sessions. Specifically, it was useful if the therapist stopped at sequences that were found to be difficult, perhaps because she felt bewildered or embarrassed, and reflected on her thoughts and feelings.

No doubt, filming of sessions will be an important tool for therapist training. The challenge is to use the concrete film as inspiration for reflection and not as a key of what actually took place. There is an obvious risk that monitoring systems like ROM and filming are being used for exercising techniques to the detriment of reflection in for instance supervision.

Skills training in relational therapy – some ideas

The exercises and tools described in the preceding section may no doubt be used in creative ways be relational therapists. They are not, however, directly focused on how to increase awareness of the therapeutic relationship.

The basic competence in relational therapy is to be reflective while in affective interaction with the patient. The challenge is to be able to let go of reflection at the right moment, to let feelings come without defensive reflection, and to regain reflectivity when the feelings are felt as imperative, as in enactments, when a third perspective is needed.

Schön (1983) argued that professionals like psychotherapists use reflection-in-action. The practitioner does not reflect, or plan, in advance. Meaningful reflections come with the professional activity. In most situations, the actual process is, however, probably stepwise rather than simultaneous. It may be more realistic to describe it as reflection-on-action, that is, reflection coming after the affective interaction (Redmond, 2006). Preparation for relational therapy would thus mean to become comfortable with fluctuations between reaction and reflection (Ensink et al., 2013).

During the session

Relational therapy is based on immediacy, spontaneity, presence. Such moments can be attended to, and in some measure trained. There are opportunities during a session when reflection about the ongoing relationship is possible. Think about how a good football team knows how to keep the ball, pass it between the players when they are uncertain about how to continue, and keep the ball on the middle ground until an opportunity emerges. This is physical image about how to wait for possibilities. In the same way, a therapist reflects on the interaction before the direction becomes clear. She talks, of course, with the patient about something that is relevant; but she has not decided what way to take. In time, a thought or an emotion will emerge that feels essential. Meanwhile, she reflects, awaits.

Outside therapy

Look at a film. Identify with one of the main persons. Try to capture his or her feelings. Try actively to decide when you would like to say something the actor does not say or do. Some films are more suitable than other. Bergman films, for instance, give great opportunities. Do the same with a novel: identify, try to capture the person's feelings. Think about what you would like to say.

Reciprocal exercises

Ask a colleague to train with you. Sit opposite each other. One of you describes an event that made a deep impression, something really moving. Think about how you react, what you want to say, what would be hard to say. Do it with eyes shut. Or let her show it with plugs in your ears.

Affect awareness

Sit alone when you read these vignettes. Try to catch what you feel. Record with your cell phone what you would like to say to the patient. Do it as self-disclosures. What do you feel, what does she feel, what do you fear saying?

"You talk with a patient that you have started appreciating. The patient talks about her fear that her boyfriend will kill himself. He is depressed and talks quite often about it. You become touched by her concerns that you perceive as realistic. The patient says: I really enjoy coming to you. No one has ever understood me the way you do. I really feel warmly about you.

"The patient has a long-term drug dependence. He has tried to quit but has never succeeded for any long time. You do not think that the patient really has any motivation and is prepared to give it up. Your picture is that the patient does not take his problems seriously and that he also treats his family in a disrespectful way. But when you met his wife once, her main concern was not his lack of respect or his abuse, it was that he had no job.

"Now you are going to tell him that either he will bring himself together or you will stop the treatment.

"Then he looks you in the eye and says that he has realized that you will never be able to help him because you have no idea what it feels like to have grown up with a dad who sometimes takes his boy into his arms and sometimes beats him and a mother who devotes herself mostly to threaten to take her life.

"You feel quite struck by his description of the difference. He is absolutely right.

"What do you say?"

When doing these exercises, be attentive on attempts at experiential avoidance. The capacity to be aware of emotions is central to therapists. Muran (2019, p. 10) quoted Billy Jean King saying: "pressure is a privilege", meaning that for therapists, it is decisive not to avoid complicated relational situations but to stay in them and try to manage them.

Training intersubjectivity

Sit together with someone you trust. One of you tells about an experience that made a strong impression. When finished, the other describes in detail how he or she feels. Compare your impressions, talk about them. Register how a way of talking and understanding, a "potential space" develops.

A caring space

Mothers do not need training to be mothers (despite the current fad for parent training). However, using the metaphorical idea that their unconscious is the first reality of the child, they need caring space for reflection. Their unconscious needs time to rest, to reflect, to grow. So do therapists. The most important for a therapist is not to train to be a good therapist, but to reflect on what kind of therapist she is.

An important way to develop is to have a fellow therapist who is ready to listen to worries, anger, shame, and bewilderment. Instead of investing money in courses in new techniques, management would do well to invest in time and space for unburdening and reflection.

In trauma therapy, therapist reactions identified as secondary traumatization have been well described (Figley & Ludick 2017). They are anxiety reactions in therapists due to confrontation with patients' narratives of extreme details of traumatic situations. This concept can be widened. All patients evoke emotional reactions, especially with engaged therapists; all therapists need ways to unburden themselves and reflect on their reactions.

Values and views of human beings

Psychotherapy is about values, about views of human life, about leading a good life. Therapists are models, or they should at least be aware that they may be seen as such (Nussbaum, 1994).

What is the perspective on a good life in relational therapy? It may be the search for a personal truth, a perspective on life grounded in reflective dialogs with significant others (Allen, 2016; Slavin, 2019). The social turbulence in recent years around truth and honesty has shown how the struggle to lead a worthy life is both social and personal. In a study of patient reactions in British primary care, Bracken et al. (2012) found that patients valued "human aspects of their encounters such as being listened to, taken seriously, and treated with dignity, kindness and respect" (p. 432) as more important than the technical expertise. Therapists need to reconcile the subjective and the professional (Åstrand & Sandell, 2019), to invite patients to become open to different views, to realize that others may carry other ideas, other perspectives (Yadlin-Gadot, 2019; Shay, 1994).

In some therapies, patients are encouraged to actively reflect on commitments to ambitions and life goals (Hayes et al., 2012). One way to get hold of one's values is to reflect on movies and novels: when you have become immersed in the action, stop and think about what values, which perspectives on the participants you share and which you dislike. Sometimes you find that people say things that surprise you, act in ways that seem hard to understand. Try to figure out what values these unexpected events indicate.

It is thought-provoking that not many years ago, curing homosexuality was seen as a reasonable goal in psychiatry and for many psychotherapists. For many, it is self-evident that the mother and not the father must be the first person who cares for the newborn child. For other, gender correction for young persons is unthinkable. The therapist's ideological beliefs are deep-seated and often unreflected, although sometimes strengthened by fitting theories. One of the gifts for the psychotherapist is that values and models of life may be challenged, if she is open for it.

Postscript

In 1934, James Strachey warned that psychoanalytic treatment might degenerate "into a real situation" (p. 146). Some critics suggest that this is what happens in relational therapy. The vital, engaged, meaningful, and serious therapeutic dialogue is assumed to create new ways of relating. Isn't that friendship?

The perspective on the interaction in therapy as mutually created and understood has radically changed the perspective of using the therapeutic relationship. It was foreboded in writings of Ferenczi and Winnicott (Berman, 2009) but matured only with the relational turn. External issues like frequency of sessions, furniture arrangements, prescribed therapist stances, have largely lost their importance when the intrinsic core of the therapeutic relationship has taken first place as change agent (Slavin, 2007a). "Not external measures, but the management of resistance and transference is the criterion for estimating whether a procedure is analysis or not" (Fenichel, 1941, p. 24). Frames and techniques do not define relational therapy; it is the creative and momentarily shaped interaction that makes treatment effective. Gradually the therapist approach has developed to a relatively spontaneous conversation. As Hoffman wrote, there are: "more times … when the conversation sounds like one that might occur in ordinary social life" (2009b, p. 624).

In parallel, psychotherapy research shows that aspects of the treatment relationship like "the real situation" (Gelso, 2009a, 2009b), therapeutic presence (Geller & Greenberg, 2012), and management of relationship troubles (Safran & Muran, 2000) have vital importance also in symptom-focused therapies. The patient's appreciation of the real relationship seems in fact to be the common factor that most strongly influences outcome (Gelso, Kivlighan, & Markin, 2018).

So, does relational therapy (and effective therapy in general) rely on the same skills and experiences as serious friendship? Or is this idea a cul-de-sac;

should therapy be a guideline-directed professional activity with clear rules and techniques, where methods can be distinguished, and outcome differences compared? Many would answer that both aspects must be there, it is the technique in combination with a constructive relationship that distinguishes therapy from friendship. Probably true, but trivial when it comes to practice.

Relational therapy contains specific interventions and a therapeutic stance. Boundaries to other methods and similarities with them may be distinguished. This perspective does not, however, give enough credit to the potential value of relational thoughts. Relational therapy implies an engaged study of an evolving helping relationship. Concepts like the third, intersubjectivity, metacommunication, potential space, and self-disclosure are not only defining characteristics of a therapy form; they are conceptual tools in ongoing studies of therapeutic relationships, potentially useful in all therapies (Slavin, 2007a).

The significance of relationality

Why would it be important to study a developing therapeutic relationship? The relational dilemma in society in our time is about independence, freedom, and loneliness in contrast to dependence, context, and intimacy. The quest for individualistic life choices, the right and possibility to choose and change life partner, job, dwelling, and, at the same time, the knowledge that we all depend on others in order to make life meaningful are the hallmarks of a modern life.

Paradoxically, we seem to move in both directions at the same time. Most people have much larger social networks than in pre-modern times. There is a contemporary trend to build networks, to create stimulating work teams and showable families. At the same time, the modern idea of training relational competencies often focuses on the individual's effort. "How to become a better lover" or "How to handle dominant leaders" are marketed on the internet. For the lone relational student.

In the psychological treatment world, there is a tendency to develop treatments based on the patient's own initiative. The patient is supposed to complete homework tasks, to make behaviour experiments, to activate himself, to meditate, to do yoga. To execute change. These treatments are effective for many patients. And foreign to relational thought.

Contemporary ideas about psychotherapeutic approaches have roots in philosophical ideas of the 19th century. In opposition to Kant, who argued that human consciousness is born from self-reflection, Hegel's idea was that human consciousness comes from recognition from the other. Subjectivity is at its root inter-subjective (Hegel, 1807: Bazzano, 2014). However, the meeting of two subjects is not uncomplicated. One subject ("thesis") meets another subject ("antithesis") and becomes vitalized through conflicts and misunderstandings. The idea that development takes place through conflicts and confrontations between persons can be applied not only on the relational, intersubjective level but also on our understanding of the social nature of mental problems. To locate them in their social and cultural context, and to find ways to approach them as social and relational problems continue to be a challenge (Sullivan, 1940).

If treatment results of cancer on the whole become more positive, there is no indication that treatment of depression and anxiety, hopelessness and irrational fear, self-destructive and self-defeating relational behaviour does. We may be certain that the view of such problems and their amelioration will differ from ours 50 years from now. But we will probably not have found ways to prevent or cure them. Mental problems are not curable; they are part of life. But they can be handled better in constructive relationships.

The position of the therapist

One of the most important consequences of the relational two-person perspective is the change in the perspective on the therapist's position. The "mutual vulnerability" (Aron, 2018) changes the therapist's authority; the patient's need to observe that the therapist changes (Slavin & Kriegman, 1998) makes therapy more personal. The contribution to the patient's development is human more than technical. It is the therapist who keeps the frame, has more experience of psychotherapy, is trained to retain the emotional focus, but in the actual interplay therapist and patient are on the same level. If the therapist's stance in traditional psychoanalysis was an extreme expression of the expert model, relational authors have turned the hands 180 degrees.

The larger perspective

The social context strongly influences our mental health. Factors like social class, employment, education, ethnicity, power position, gender, sex, and age frame our possibilities to get psychotherapy and to benefit from it (Gentile, 2017; Layton et al., 2006). The neoliberal ideology, the idea that there are limitless choices and limitless personal responsibility for success and failure, is probably a significant cause for contemporary mental unhealth (Layton, 2018).

Psychoanalysis as a theory, and the knowledge gained from psychoanalytic treatments, have had a large influence on the scientific and cultural understanding of human predicaments. Although Freud was uninterested in politics, his theory early drew attention as a radical critique of conventional bourgeois views, particularly regarding sexual attitudes. Later, psychoanalysts have recurrently taken radical stands on political issues, fighting for liberal views on social questions (Jacoby, 1986). It is an open question to what extent the relational movement will influence culture and society more generally. The relational tradition grew out of the cultural and political upheavals in the 1960s and 1970s (Safran, 2017). Relational authors have been outspoken against the misuse of concepts like knowledge and truth among populist politicians (Jurist, 2018; Fonagy & Allison, 2015). Davies (2019) pointed to the similarity between the lies and crimes of President Trump and his accomplices, and the experiences of molested and abused children. We are the victims of perpetrators, persons who can get away with anything, of idealized saviors, to whom we unrealistically and naively fix our expectations, and to unseeing witnesses who let their comfort and position trump their conscience.

The journey through some aspects of relational theory, set in relation to empirical findings, has shown its creativity and vitality. It may be important to not just return to where it came from but to head towards rewarding contacts with the rest of the psychotherapy world.

References

Aafjes-Van Doorn, K., & Barber, J. P. (2017). Systematic review of in-session affect experience in cognitive behavioral therapy for depression. *Cognitive Therapy and Research, 41*, 807–828.

Ainsworth, M. D. S., Blehar, M. C., Waters, E., & Wall, S. (1978). *Patterns of attachment: A psychological study of the strange situation.* Hillsdale, NJ: Lawrence Erlbaum.

Albani, C., Benninghofen, D., Blaser, G., Cierpka, M., Dahlbender, R., Geyer, M., et al. (1999). On the connection between affective evaluation of recollected relationship experiences and the severity of the psychic impairment. *Psychotherapy Research, 9*, 452–467.

Alexander, F., & French, T. (1946). *Psycho-analytic therapy.* New York: Ronald Press.

Alfi-Yogev, T., Hasson-Ohayon, I., Lazarus, G., Ziv-Beiman, S., & Atzil-Slonim, D. (2020) When to disclose and to whom? examining within- and between-client moderators of therapist self-disclosure – outcome associations in psychodynamic psychotherapy. *Psychotherapy Research* (advance online publication).

Allen, J. G. (2016). Should the century-old practice of psychotherapy defer to science and ignore its foundations in two millenia of ethical thought? *Bulletin of the Menninger Clinic, 80*, 1–29.

Allen, J. G., Fonagy, P., & Bateman, A. (2008). *Mentalizing in clinical practice.* Arlington, VA: American Psychiatric Association.

Allison, E., & Fonagy, P. (2016). When is truth relevant? *Psychoanalytic Quarterly, 85*(1), 275–303.

Amble, I., Gude, T., Stubdal, S., Andersen, B. J., & Wampold, B. E. (2015). The effect of implementing the Outcome Questionnaire-45.2 feedback system in Norway: A multisite randomized clinical trial in a naturalistic setting. *Psychotherapy Research, 25*, 669–677.

American Psychological Association Presidential Task Force on Evidence-Based Practice. (2006). Evidence-based practice in psychology. *American Psychologist, 61*, 271–285.

Anderson, T., Crowley, M. E. J., Himawan, L., Holmberg, J. K., & Uhlin, B. D. (2016a). Therapist facilitative interpersonal skills and training status: A randomized clinical trial on alliance and outcome. *Psychotherapy Research, 26*, 511–529.

Anderson, T., McClintock, A. S., Himawan, L., Song, X., & Patterson, C. L. (2016b). A prospective study of therapist facilitative interpersonal skills as a predictor of treatment outcome. *Journal of Consulting and Clinical Psychology*, *84*, 57–66.

Antaki, C. (2008). Formulations in psychotherapy. In A. Peräkylä (Ed.), *Conversation analysis and psychotherapy* (pp. 26–42). Cambridge: Cambridge University Press.

Antaki, C., Barnes, R., & Leudar I. (2005). Self-disclosure as a situated interactional practice. *British Journal of Social Psychology*, *44*, 1–20.

Aragno, A. (2008). The language of empathy: An analysis of its constitution, development, and role in psychoanalytic listening. *Journal of the American Psychoanalytic Association*, *56*, 713–740.

Aron, L. (1996). *A meeting of minds*. Hillsdale, NJ: The Analytic Press.

Aron, L. (1999). Clinical choices and the relational matrix. *Psychoanalytic Dialogues*, *9*, 1–29.

Aron, L. (2006), Analytic impasse and the third: Clinical implications of inter-subjectivity theory. *International Journal of Psycho-Analysis*, *87*, 349–368.

Aron. L. (2014). "With you I'm Born Again": Themes and fantasies of birth and the family circumstances surrounding birth as these are mutually evoked in patient and analyst. *Psychoanalytic Dialogues*, *24*, 341–357.

Aron, L. (2018). Beyond tolerance in psychoanalytic communities. In L. Aron, S. Grand, & J. Slochower (Eds.), *Decentering relational theory. A comparative critique*. London: Routledge.

Aron, L., & Atlas, G. (2015). Generative enactment: Memories from the future. *Psychoanalytic Dialogues*, *25*, 309–324.

Aron, L., Grand, S., & Slochower, J. (2018a). *De-idealizing relational theory. A critique from within*. London: Routledge.

Aron, L., Grand, S., & Slochower, J. (2018b). *Decentering relational theory. A comparative critique*. London: Routledge.

Aron, L., & Leichich, M. (2012) Relational psychoanalysis. In: G. Gabbard, B. Litowitz, & P. Williams (Eds.), *Textbook of psychoanalysis* (2nd ed.). Arlington, VA: American Psychiatric Publishing.

Åstrand, K., & Sandell, R. (2019). Influence of personal therapy on learning and development of psychotherapeutic skills. *Psychoanalytic Psychotherapy*, *33*, 34–48.

Atzil-Slonim, D., & Tschacher, W. (2020). Dynamic dyadic processes in psychotherapy: Introduction to a special section. *Psychotherapy Research*, *30*, 555–557.

Averill, J. R. (2012). The future of social constructionism: Introduction to a special section of emotion review. *Emotion Review*, *4*, 215–220.

Bach, S. (2006). *Getting from here to there*. Hillsdale, NJ: Analytic Press.

Baker, T. B., & McFall, R. M. (2014). The promise of science-based training and application in psychological clinical science. *Psychotherapy*, *51*, 482–486.

Balint, M. (1968). *The basic fault*. London: Tavistock.

Baldwin, M. (2000). Interview with Carl Rogers on the use of the self in therapy. In I. M. Baldwin (Ed.), *The use of self in therapy* (2nded., pp. 29–38). New York: Haworth Press.

Baranger, M., & Baranger, W. (2008). The analytic situation as a dynamic field. *The International Journal of Psychoanalysis*, *89*, 795–826 (Original work published 1961–1962).

Baranger, M., Baranger, W., & Mom, J. (1983). Process and non-process in analytic work. *International Journal of Psycho-Analysis*, *64*, 1–15.

Barber, J., Muran, C., McCarthy, K., & Keefe, J. (2013). Research on dynamic therapies. In *Bergin and Garfield's handbook of psychotherapy and behavior change* (6th ed., pp. 443–494). New York, NY: John Wiley & Sons.

Barlow, D. H. (2004). Psychological treatments. *American Psychologist, 59*, 869–878.

Barlow, D. H., & Farchione, T. J. (2017). *Applications of the unified protocol for transdiagnostic treatment of emotional disorders.* New York, NY: Oxford University Press.

Barlow, D. H., & Kennedy, K. A. (2016). New approaches to diagnosis and treatment in anxiety and related emotional disorders: A focus on temperament. *Canadian Psychology/Psychologie canadienne, 57*, 8–20.

Barreto, J. F., Nata, G., & Matos, P. M. (2020). Elaboration of countertransference experience and the workings of the working alliance. *Psychotherapy, 57*, 141–150.

Barrett, L. F. (2017). *How emotions are made: The secret life of the brain.* New York, NY: Houghton Mifflin Harcourt.

Bass, A. (2014). Three pleas for a measure of uncertainty, reverie, and private contemplation in the chaotic, interactive, nonlinear dynamic field of interpersonal/ intersubjective relational psychoanalysis. *Psychoanalytic Dialogues, 24*, 663–675.

Bateman, A., Campbell, C., Luyten, P., & Fonagy, P. (2017). A mentalization-based approach to common factors in the treatment of borderline personality disorder. *Current Opinion in Psychology, 21*, 44–49.

Bateman, A. W., & Fonagy, P. (2006). *Mentalization-based treatment for borderline personality disorder.* Oxford: Oxford University Press.

Bateman, A., & Fonagy, P. (2012). *Handbook of mentalizing in mental health practice.* Arlington, VA: American Psychiatric Publishing.

Bateman, A., & Fonagy, P. (2016). *Mentalization-based treatment for personality disorders: A practical guide.* Oxford: Oxford University Press.

Baumann, Z. (2000). Liquid Modernity. Cambridge: Polity.

Bazzano, M. (2014). Togetherness: intersubjectivity revisited. *Person-Centered & Experiential Psychotherapies, 13*, 203–216.

Beck, U., & Beck-Gernsheim, E. (2002). *Individualization. Institutionalized individualism and its social and political consequences.* London: Sage.

Beebe, B., Jaffe, J., Markese, S., Buck, K., Chen, H., Cohen, P., … Feldstein, S. (2010). The origins of 12-month attachment: A microanalysis of 4-month mother-infant interaction. *Attachment & Human Development, 12*, 2–141.

Beebe, B., Knoblauch, S., Rustin, J., & Sorter, D. (2005). *Forms of intersubjectivity in infant research and adult treatment.* New York, NY: Other press.

Beebe, B., & Lachmann, F. (1994), Representation and internalization in infancy: Three principles of salience. *Psychoanalytic. Psychology, 11*, 127–165.

Beebe, B., & Lachmann, F. (2013). *The origins of attachment: Infant research and adult treatment.* New York: Routledge Press.

Beebe, B., & Lachmann, F. (2020). Infant research and adult treatment revisited: Cocreating self- and interactive regulation. *Psychoanalytic Psychology, 37*, 313–323.

Beebe, B., Lachmann, F., Markese, S., Buck, K.A., Bahrick, LE, Chen, H, … Jaffe, J. (2012). On the origins of disorganized attachment and internal working models: Paper II. An empirical microanalysis of 4-month mother-infant interaction. *Psychoanalytic Dialogues, 22*(3), 352–374.

Beebe, B., Jaffe, J., & Lachmann, F. M. (1992). A dyadic systems view of communication. In N. Skolnick & S. C. Warshaw (Eds.), *Relational perspectives in psychoanalysis*. New York: The Analytic Press.

Beebe, B., Rustin, J., Sorter, D., & Knoblauch, S. (2003). An expanded view of intersubjectivity in infancy and its application to psychoanalysis. *Psychoanalytic Dialogues, 13*, 805–841.

Benish, S. G., Imel, Z. E., & Wampold, B. E. (2008). The relative efficacy of bona fide psychotherapies for treating post-traumatic stress disorder: A meta-analysis of direct comparisons. *Clinical Psychology Review, 28*, 746–758.

Benjamin J. (1988). *The bonds of love: Psychoanalysis, feminism, and the problem of domination*. New York, NY: Pantheon.

Benjamin, J. (1990). An outline of intersubjectivity: The development of recognition. *Psychoanalytic Psychology, 7*, 33–46.

Benjamin, J. (1995). *Like subjects, love objects: Essays on recognition and sexual difference*. NY: Yale University Press.

Benjamin, L. S. (1996). *Interpersonal diagnosis and treatment of personality disorders*. New York: The Guilford Press.

Benjamin, J. (2004). Beyond doer and done to: An intersubjective view of thirdness. *The Psychoanalytic Quarterly, 73*, 5–46.

Benjamin, J. (2007). Listening together: Intersubjective aspects of the analytic process of losing and restoring recognition. In S. Akhtar (Ed.), *Listening to others: Developmental and clinical aspects of empathy and attunement*. NY: Jason Aronson.

Benjamin, J. (2017). *Beyond doer and done to: Recognition theory, intersubjectivity*. London and New York: Routledge.

Bennett-Levy, J. (2019). Why therapists should walk the talk: The theoretical and empirical case for personal practice in therapist training and professional development. *Journal of Behavior Therapy and Experimental Psychiatry, 62*, 133–145.

Berman, E. (2009). Ferenczi and Winnicott: Why we need their radical edge: Commentary on paper by Michael Parsons. *Psychoanalytic Dialogues, 19*, 246–252.

Bernhardt, I. S., Nissen-Lie, H. A., & Råbu, M. (2020). The embodied listener: A dyadic case study of how therapist and patient reflect on the significance of therapist's personal presence for the therapeutic change process. *Psychotherapy Research*, ahead-of-print, 1–13.

Bernstein, J. (1999), Countertransference: Our new royal road to the unconscious? *Psychoanalytic Dialogues, 9*, 275–299.

Beutler, L. E., Kimpara, S., Edwards, C. J., Miller, K. D. (2018). Fitting psychotherapy to patient coping style: A meta-analysis. *Journal of Clinical Psychology, 74*, 1980–1995.

Binder, J., & Strupp, H. (1997). "Negative process": A recurrently discovered and underestimated facet of therapeutic process and outcome in the individual psychotherapy of adults. *Clinical Psychology: Science and Practice, 4*, 121–139.

Bion, W. R. (1962). *Learning from experience*. London: William Heinemann.

Bion, W. R. (1967). *Second thoughts*. London: William Heinemann.

218   *References*

Bion, W. R. (1970). *Attention and interpretation: A scientific approach to insight in psycho-analysis and groups*. London, UK: Tavistock.
Black, Margaret J.(2003). Enactment: Analytic musings on energy, language, and personal growth. *Psychoanalytic Dialogues, 13*, 633–655.
Blum, H. P. (2003). Repression, transference and reconstruction. *International Journal of Psychoanalysis, 84*, 497–503.
Bohart, A. C. (1991). Empathy in client-centered therapy: A contrast with psycho-analysis and self psychology. *Journal of Humanistic Psychology, 31*, 34–48.
Bohart, A. C. (2000). The client is the most important common factor: Clients' self-healing capacities and psychotherapy. *Journal of Psychotherapy Integration, 10*, 127–149.
Bollas, C. (1987). *The shadow of the object*. London, UK: Free Association Books
Bollas, C. (2015). An Interview with Arne Jemstedt. *International Forum of Psychoanalysis, 24*, 182–188.
Bolognini S. (1997). Empathy and 'empathism'. *International Journal of Psychoanalysis, 78*, 279–293.
Bordin, E. S. (1994). Theory and research on the therapeutic working alliance: New directions. In A. O. Horvath & L. S. Greenberg (Eds.), *The working alliance: Theory, research, and practice*. New York, NY: Wiley.
Boston Change Process Study Group. (2002). Explicating the implicit: the local level and the microprocess of change in the analytic situation. *International Journal of Psychoanalysis, 83*, 1051–1062.
Boston Change Process Study Group. (2010). *Change in Psychotherapy: A Unifying Paradigm*. New York: W. W. Norton.
Boston Change Process Study Group. (2018a). Engagement and the emergence of a charged other. *Contemporary Psychoanalysis, 54*, 540–559.
Boston Change Process Study Group. (2018b). Moving through and being moved by: Embodiment in development and in the therapeutic relationship. *Contemporary Psychoanalysis, 54*, 299–321.
Bowlby, J. (1969). *Attachment and loss, Volume 1: Attachment*. New York: Basic Books.
Bowlby, J. (1988). *A secure base: Parent–child attachment and healthy human development*. New York, NY: Basic Books.
Bracken, P., Thomas, P., Timimi, S., Asen, E., Behr, G., Beuster, C., et al. (2012). Psychiatry beyond the current paradigm. *British Journal of Psychiatry, 201*, 430–434.
Bram, A. D. & Gabbard, G. O. (2001). Potential space and reflective functioning: Towards conceptual clarification and preliminary clinical implications. *The International Journal of Psychoanalysis, 82*, 685–699.
Brazelton, T. B., B. Kozlowski, & M. Main. (1974), The origins of reciprocity: The early mother–infant interaction. In M. Lewis & R. Rosenblum (Eds.), *The effect of the infant on its caretaker*. New York: Wiley.
Brenner, C. (1968). Psychoanalysis and science. *Journal of the American Psychoanalytic Association, 16*, 675–696.
Brenner, C. (1982). *The mind in conflict*. NY: International Universities Press.
Bressi, C., Fronza, S., Minacapelli, E., Nocito, E. P., Dipasquale, E., Magri, L., … Barone, L. (2017). Short-term psychodynamic psychotherapy with mentalization-based techniques in major depressive disorder patients: Relationship among

alexithymia, reflective functioning, and outcome variables – a pilot study. *Psychology and Psychotherapy*, *90*, 299–313. Frank Lachmann.

Breuer, J., & Freud, S. (1895). *Studien über Hysterie.* Wien: Franz Deuticke.

Briere, J. (1997). Treating adults severely abused as children: The self-trauma model. In D. A. Wolfe, R. J. McMahon, & R. D. Peters (Eds.), *Child abuse: New directions in prevention and treatment across the lifespan.* Thousand Oaks, CA: Sage Inc.

Briere, J., Agee, E., & Dietrich, A. (2016). Cumulative trauma and current post-traumatic stress disorder status in general population and inmate samples. *Psychological Trauma: Theory, Research, Practice, and Policy*, *8*, 439–446.

Bromberg, P. M. (1993). Shadow and substance: A relational perspective on clinical process. In P. M. Bromberg (Ed.), *Standing in the spaces: Essays on clinical process, trauma, and dissociation.* Hillsdale, NJ: The Analytic Press.

Bromberg, P. (1998). *Standing in the spaces: Essays on dissociation, trauma, and clinical process.* Hillsdale, NJ: The Analytic Press.

Bromberg, P. (2006). *Awakening the dreamer: Clinical journeys.* Hillsdale, NJ: The Analytic Press.

Bromberg, P. M. (2011). *The shadow of the Tsunami: And the growth of the relational mind.* New York, NY: Routledge.

Bromberg, P. M. (2012a). Stumbling along and hanging in: If this be technique, make the most of it. *Psychoanalytic Inquiry*, *32*, 3–17.

Bromberg, P. (2012b). Credo. *Psychoanalytic dialogues*, *22*, 273–278.

Bruner, J. (1990), *Acts of meaning.* Cambridge, MA: Havard University Press.

Buber, M. (1923). *Ich und Du.* Leipzig: Inter Verlag. English translation I and Thou (1970). New York: Touchstone.

Buber, M. (1946). *Between man and man.* London:Routledge.

Bucci, W. (1997). *Psychoanalysis and cognitive science: A multiple code theory.* NY: Guilford Press.

Bucci, W. (2011). The interplay of subsymbolic and symbolic processes in psycho-analytic treatment: It takes two to tango—But who knows the steps, who's the leader? The choreography of psychoanalytic interchange. *Psychoanalytic Dialogues*, *21*, 45–54.

Bucci, W. (2018). The primary process as a transitional concept: New perspectives from cognitive psychology and affective neuroscience. *Psychoanalytic Inquiry*, *38*, 198–209.

Busch, F. (2010). Distinguishing psychoanalysis from psychotherapy. *International Journal of Psychoanalysis*, *91*, 23–34.

Busch, F. (2014). *Creating a psychoanalytic mind: A psychoanalytic method and theory.* London: Routledge/Taylor & Francis Group.

Cacioppo, J. T., & Berntson, G. G. (1992). Social psychological contributions to the decade of the brain: Doctrine of multilevel analysis. *American Psychologist*, *47*, 1019–1028.

Cacioppo, J. T., Cacioppo, S., & Dulawa, S. (2014). Social neuroscience and its potential contribution to psychiatry. *World Psychiatry*, *13*, 131–139.

Calhoun, L. (1995). The philosophy of discreditation: An essay on actuality and possibility. *Journal of Social Philosophy*, *26*, 66–72.

Caspi, A., & Moffitt, T. E. (2018). All for one and one for all: Mental disorders in one dimension. *American Journal of Psychiatry*, *175*, 831– 844.

220   *References*

Castonguay, L. G., & Hill, C. E. (Eds.). (2012). *Transformation in psychotherapy: Corrective experiences across cognitive behavioral, humanistic, and psychodynamic approaches.* Washington: American Psychological Association.

Chambless, D. L., Sanderson, W. C., Shoham, V., Bennett Johnson, S., Pope, K.S., Crits-Christoph, P., ... McCurry, S. (1996). An update on empirically validated therapies. *The Clinical Psychologist, 49,* 5–18.

Chefetz, R. A., & Bromberg, P. M. (2004). Talking with "Me" and "Not-Me": A dialogue. *Contemporary Psychoanalysis, 40,* 409–464.

Chen, R., Atzil-Slonim, D., Bar-Kalifa, E., Hasson-Ohayon, I., & Refaeli, E. (2018). Therapists' recognition of alliance ruptures as a moderator of change in alliance and symptoms. *Psychotherapy Research, 28,* 560–570.

Chow, D. L., Miller, S. D., Seidel, J. A., Kane, R. T., Thornton, J. A., & Andrews, W. P. (2015). The role of deliberate practice in the development of highly effective psychotherapists. *Psychotherapy, 52,* 337–345.

Chui, H., Hill, C. E., Kline, K., Kuo, P., & Mohr, J. J. (2016). Are you in the mood? Therapist affect and psychotherapy process. *Journal of Counseling Psychology, 63,* 405–418.

Cierpka, M., Strack, M., Benninghoven, D., Staats, H., Dahlbender, R., Pokorny, D., et al. (1998). Stereotypical relationship patterns and psychopathology. *Psychotherapy & Psychosomatics, 67,* 241–248.

Clemen, G. (1997). The concept of hedging: Origins, approaches and definitions. In R. Markkanen & H. Schröder (Eds.), *Hedging and discourse. Approaches to the analysis of a pragmatic phenomenon in academic texts.* Berlin: Walter de Gruyter.

Colli, A., Tanzilli, A., Dimaggio, G., & Lingiardi, V. (2014). Patient personality and therapist response: An empirical investigation. *American Journal of Psychiatry, 171,* 102–108.

Cologon, J., Schweitzer, R. D., King, R., & Nolte, T. (2017). Therapist reflective functioning, therapist attachment style and therapist effectiveness. *Administration and Policy in Mental Health, 44,* 614–625.

Cooney, A. S. (2018). Vitalizing enactment: A relational exploration. *Psychoanalytic Dialogues, 28,* 340–354.

Cooper, S. (2008), Privacy, reverie, and the analyst's ethical imagination. *Psychoanalytic Quarterly, 77,* 1045–1073.

Cooper, S. (2010). *Disturbance in the field. Essays in transference-countertransference.* London: Routledge.

Cooper, M. (2019). *Integrating counselling and psychotherapy. Directionality, synergy, and social change.* SAGE.

Cornelius, J. T. (2018). The case for psychoanalysis: Exploring the scientific evidence. In R. E. Barsness (Ed.), *Core competencies of relational psychoanalysis: A guide to practice, study, and research.* London: Routledge.

Crane, R. S., Brewer, J., Feldman, C., Kabat-Zinn, J., Santorelli, S., Williams, J. M. G., & Kuyken, W. (2017). What defines mindfulness-based programs? The warp and the weft. *Psychological Medicine, 47,* 990–999.

Crits-Christoph, P., Barber, J. P., & Kurcias, J. S. (1993). The accuracy of therapists' interpretations and the development of the therapeutic alliance. *Psychotherapy Research, 3,* 25–35.

Crits-Christoph, P., & Gibbons, M. B. C. (2002). Relational interpretations. In J. C. Norcross, (Ed.), *Psychotherapy relationships that work: Therapist contributions and responsiveness to patients.* London: Oxford University Press.

Cromer, T. D., & Hilsenroth, M. J. (2010). Patient personality and outcome in short-term psychodynamic psychotherapy. *Journal of Nervous and Mental Disease, 198,* 59–66.

Cuijpers P. (2016). Are all psychotherapies equally effective in the treatment of adult depression? The lack of statistical power of comparative outcome studies. *Evidence Based Mental Health, 19,* 39–42.

Cuijpers, P., Karyotaki, E., Reijnders, M., & Ebert, D. D. (2018). Was Eysenck right after all? A reassessment of the effects of psychotherapy for adult depression. *Epidemiology and Psychiatric Sciences, 28,* 21–30.

Cuijpers, P., Reijnders, M., & Huibers, M. J. H. (2019). The role of common factors in psychotherapy outcomes. *Annual Review of Clinical Psychology,* 15, 207–231.

Cushman, P. (1996). *Constructing the selfs: Constructing America: A cultural history of psychotherapy.* Cambridge, MA: DaCapo Press.

Dahl, H.-S. J., Røssberg, J.I., Crits-Christoph, P., Gabbard, G.O., Hersoug, A.G., Perry, J.J., Ulberg, R., & Høglend, P. (2014). Long-term effects of analysis of the patient therapist relationship in the context of patients' personality pathology and therapists' parental feelings. *Journal of Consulting and Clinical Psychology, 82,* 460–471.

Dahl, H. S., Ulberg, R., Friis, S., Perry, J. C., & Høglend, P. A. (2016). Therapists' inadequate feelings and long-term effect of transference work. *Psychotherapy and Psychosomatics, 85,* 309–310.

Damasio, A. (1999). *The feeling of what happens: Body and emotion in the making of consciousness.* New York, NY: Norton.

Damasio, A. (2010). *Self comes to mind: Constructing the conscious brain.* New York: Pantheon/Random House.

Daniel, S. I. F. (2015). *Adult attachment patterns in a treatment context: Relationship and narrative.* London: Routledge/Taylor & Francis Group.

Davanloo, H. (1995). *Unlocking the unconscious: Selected papers of Habib Davanloo.* New York: John Wiley & Sons.

Davies, J. M. (1999). Getting cold feet, defining "safe enough" borders: Dissociation, multiplicity, and integration in the analyst's experience. *The Psychoanalytic Quarterly, LXVIII,* 184–208.

Davies, J. M. (2003). Falling in love with love: Oedipal and postoedipal manifestations of idealization, mourning and erotic masochism. *Psychoanalytic Dialogues, 13,* 1–27.

Davies, J. M. (2016). The man who would be everything (to everyone): The unconscious realities and fantasies of psychic truth and change. *The Psychoanalytic Quarterly, 85,* 361–391.

Davies, J. M. (2018). The 'once and future' focus of a relational psychoanalysis: Discussion of 'vitalizing enactment'. *Psychoanalytic Dialogues, 28,* 355–360.

Davies, J. M. (2018). The "rituals" of the relational perspective: Theoretical shifts and clinical implications. *Psychoanalytic Dialogues, 28,* 651–669.

Davies, J. M. (2019) Truth and consequence: Alternative facts and discordant realities. *Psychoanalytic Dialogues, 29,* 165–171.

Davies, J. M., & Frawley, M. G. (1992). Dissociative processes and transference-countertransference paradigms in the psychoanalytically oriented treatment of adult survivors of childhood sexual abuse. *Psychoanalytic Dialogues, 2,* 5–36.

Davis, K. (1986). The process of problem (re)formulation in psychotherapy. *Sociology of Health & Illness, 8,* 44–74.

de Felice, G., Giuliani, A., Halfon, S., Andreassi, S., Paoloni, G., & Orsucci, F. F. (2019). The misleading Dodo Bird verdict. How much of the outcome variance is explained by common and specific factors? *New Ideas in Psychology, 54,* 50–55.

de Jong, K., van Sluis, P., Nugter, M. A., Heiser, W. J., & Spinhoven, P. (2012). Understanding the differential impact of outcome monitoring: Therapist variables that moderate feedback effects in a randomized clinical trial. *Psychotherapy Research, 22,* 464–474.

De Peyer, J. (2016). Uncanny communication and the porous mind. *Psychoanalytic Dialogues, 26,* 156–174.

DeFife, J. A., Hilsenroth, M. J., & Kuutmann, K. (2015). Beyond transference: Fostering growth through therapeutic immediacy. In P. Luyten, L. C. Mayes, P. Fonagy, M. Target, & S. Blatt (Eds.), *Handbook of psychodynamic approaches to psychopathology.* London: The Guilford Press.

Delgadillo, J., de Jong, K., Lucock, M., Lutz, W., Rubel, J., Gilbody, S., ... McMillan, D. (2018). Feedback-informed treatment versus usual psychological treatment for depression and anxiety: A multisite, open-label, cluster randomised controlled trial. *The Lancet Psychiatry, 5,* 564–572.

Del Re, A. C., Flückiger, C., Horvath, A. O., & Wampold, B. E. (2021). Examining therapist effects in the alliance–outcome relationship: A multilevel meta-analysis. *Journal of Consulting and Clinical Psychology, 89,* 371–378.

DiAmbrosio, P. E. (2014). Patient and analyst in crises: A mutual transformation reflected in a clinical narrative and St. Exupery's 'The little prince'. *International Journal of Psychoanalytic Self Psychology, 9,* 131–143.

Diamond, D., Stovall-McClough, C., Clarkin, J. F., & Levy, K. N. (2003). Patient-therapist attachment in the treatment of borderline personality disorder. *Bulletin of the Menninger Clinic, 67,* 227–259.

Dinger, U., Zilcha-Mano, S., McCarthy, K. S., Barrett, M. S., & Barber, J. P. (2013). Interpersonal problems as predictors of alliance, symptomatic improvement and premature termination in treatment of depression. *Journal of Affective Disorders, 151,* 800–803.

Director, L. (2016). The analyst as catalyst: Cultivating mind in the shadow of neglect. *Psychoanalytic Dialogues, 26,* 685–697.

Downing, G. (2006). Early affect change and the body. In G. Marlock & H. Weiss (Eds.), *Handbuch der Körperpsychotherapie [Handbook of body-oriented psychotherapy].* Göttingen: Hogreve.

Driessen, E., Hegelmaier, L. M., Abbass, A. A., Barber, J. P., Dekker, J. J.M., Van, H. L., Jansma, E. P., & Cuijpers, P. (2015). The efficacy of short-term psychodynamic psychotherapy for depression: A meta-analysis update. Clinical Psychology Review, 42, 1–15.

Drozek, R. (2015). The dignity in multiplicity: Human value as a foundational concept in relational thought. *Psychoanalytic Dialogues, 25,* 431–451.

Duarte, J., Martinez, C., & Tomicic, A. (2020). Episodes of meeting in psychotherapy: An empirical exploration of patients' experiences of subjective change during their psychotherapy process. *Research in Psychotherapy: Psychopathology, Process and Outcome, 23*, 56–66.

Ehrenberg, D. B. (1992). *The Intimate Edge*. New York: Norton.

Ekeblad, A., Falkenström, F., & Holmqvist, R. (2016). Reflective functioning as predictor of working alliance and outcome in the treatment of depression. *Journal of Consulting and Clinical Psychology, 84*, 67–78.

Ekman, P. (1992). An argument for basic emotions. *Cognition and Emotion, 6*, 169–200.

Ekman, P., Campos, J. J., Davidson, R. J., & de Wall, F. B. M. (Eds.). (2003). *Emotions inside out: 130 years after Darwin's The Expression of the Emotions in Man and Animals (Annals of the New York Academy of Sciences, Vol. 1000)*. New York: New York Academy of Sciences. Ellsworth, P. C. (2013). Appraisal theory: Old and new questions. *Emotion Review, 5*, 125–131.

Ellsworth, P. C. (2013). Appraisal theory: Old and new questions. *Emotion Review, 5*, 125–131.

Ensink, K., Maheux, J., Normandin, L., Sabourin, S., Diguer, L., Berthelot, N., & Parent, K. (2013). The impact of mentalization training on the reflective function of novice therapists: A randomized controlled trial. *Psychotherapy Research, 23*, 526–553.

Ericsson, K. A. (2009). Enhancing the development of professional performance: Implications from the study of deliberate practice. In K. A. Ericsson (Ed.), *Development of professional expertise: Toward measurement of expert performance and design of optimal learning environments* (pp. 405–431). New York, NY: Cambridge University Press.

Ericsson, K. A., Krampe, R. T., & Tesch-Romer, C. (1993). The role of deliberate practice in the acquisition of expert performance. *Psychological Review, 100*, 363–406.

Eriksson, T., Germundsjö, L., Åström, E., & Rönnlund, M. (2018). Mindful self-compassion training reduces stress and burnout symptoms among practicing psychologists: A randomized controlled trial of a brief web-based intervention. *Frontiers in Psychology, 9*, 1–10.

Etchegoyen, R. H. (1991). *The fundamentals of psychoanalytic technique*. London: Taylor and Francis.

Eubanks, C., Muran, C., & Safran, J. (2019). Repairing alliance ruptures. In J. Norcross & M. Lambert (Eds.), *Psychotherapy relationships that work* (pp. 549–579). New York, NY: Oxford University Press.

Eubanks-Carter, C., Muran, J. C., & Safran, J. D. (2015). Alliance-focused training. *Psychotherapy, 52*, 169–173.

Fairbairn, W. R. D. (1952). *Psychoanalytic Studies of the Personality*. London: Routledge & Kegan Paul.

Falkenström, F. (2007). The psychodynamics of self-observation. *Psychoanalytic Dialogues, 17*, 551–574.

Falkenström, F., Ekeblad, A., & Holmqvist, R. (2016). Improvement of the working alliance in one treatment session predicts improvement of depressive symptoms by the next session. *Journal of Consulting and Clinical Psychology, 84*, 738– 751.

Falkenström, F. & Holmqvist, R. (2021). "Therapist In-Session Feelings Predict Change in Depressive Symptoms in Interpersonal and Brief Relational Psychotherapy" It is not manuscript, it is "advance online publication".

Falkenström, F., Josefsson, A., Berggren, T., & Holmqvist, R. (2016). How much therapy is enough? Comparing dose-effect and good-enough models in two different settings. *Psychotherapy, 53*, 130–139

Fearon, P., Y. Shmueli-Goetz, E. Viding, P. Fonagy, & R. Plomin. (2014), Genetic and environmental influences on adolescent attachment. *Journal of Child Psychology and Psychiatry, 55*, 1033–1041.

Fenichel, O. (1941). *Problems of psychoanalytic technique* [Trans. by D. Brunswick]. Psychoanalytic Quarterly, Inc.

Ferenczi, S. (1928). The elasticity of psychoanalytic technique. In J. Borossa (Ed.), 1999. *Selected writings of Sandor Ferenczi*. London: Penguin.

Ferenczi, S. (1933) A confusion of tongues between adults and the child. In J. Borossa (Ed.), 1999. *Selected writings of Sandor Ferenczi*. London: Penguin.

Ferro, A. (2011). Clinical implications of Bion's thought. In C. Mawson (Ed.), *Bion today*. London: Routledge/Taylor & Francis Group.

Figley, C. R. & Ludick, M. (2017). Secondary traumatization and compassion fatigue. In S. N. Gold (Ed.), *APA handbook of trauma psychology: Foundations in knowledge*. Washington: American Psychological Association.

Flückiger, C., Del Re, A. C., Wampold, B. E., & Horvath, A. O. (2018). The alliance in adult psychotherapy: A meta-analytic synthesis. *Psychotherapy, 55*, 316–340.

Flückiger, C., Del Re, A. C., Wlodasch, D., Horvath, A. O., Solomonov, N., & Wampold, B. E. (2020). Assessing the alliance–outcome association adjusted for patient characteristics and treatment processes: A meta-analytic summary of direct comparisons. *Journal of Counseling Psychology, 67*, 706–711.

Foa, E.B., Hembree, E.A., Rothbaum, B.O., & Rach, S.A.M. (2019). *Prolonged exposure therapy for PTSD*. Oxford University Press.

Fosha, D. (2000). *The transforming power of affect*. New York: Basic Books.

Fosha, D., Thoma, N., & Yeung, D. (2019). Transforming emotional suffering into flourishing: metatherapeutic processing of positive affect as a trans-theoretical vehicle for change. *Counselling Psychology Quarterly, 32*, 563–593.

Fonagy, P. (1999). Memory and therapeutic action (guest editorial). *International Journal of Psychoanalysis, 80*, 215–223.

Fonagy, P. (1999). Relation of theory and practice in psychodynamic therapy. *Journal of Clinical Child Psychology, 28*(4), 513–520.

Fonagy, P. (2010). Psychotherapy research: Do we know what works for whom? *The British Journal of Psychiatry: The Journal of Mental Science, 197*, 83–85.

Fonagy, P., & Allison, E. (2014). The role of mentalizing and epistemic trust in the therapeutic relationship. *Psychotherapy, 51*, 372–380.

Fonagy, P. Allison, E., & Campbell, C. (2019) Commentary on "'Trust comes from a sense of feeling one's self understood by another mind': An interview with Peter Fonagy". *Psychoanalytic Psychology, 36*, 228.

Fonagy, P & Campbell, C. (2015). Bad blood revisited: Attachment and psychoanalysis. *British Journal of Psychotherapy 31*, 229–250.

Fonagy, P., Edgcumbe, R., Moran, G. S., Kennedy, H., & Target, M. (1993). The roles of mental representations and mental processes in therapeutic action. *Psychoanalytic Study of the Child, 48*, 9–48.

Fonagy, P., Gergely, G., Jurist, E., & Target, M. (2002). *Affect regulation, mentalization and the development of the self*. New York, NY: Other Press.

Fonagy, P., Gergely, G., Jurist, E., & Target, M. (2005). *Affect regulation, mentalization, and the development of the self*. London: Karnac.

Fonagy, P., Gergely, G., & Target, M. (2007). The parent–infant dyad and the construction of the subjective self. *Journal* of *Child Psychology and Psychiatry, 48*, 288–328.

Fonagy, P., Luyten, P., & Allison, E. (2015). Epistemic petrification and the restoration of epistemic trust: A new conceptualization of borderline personality disorder and its psychosocial treatment. *Journal of Personality Disorders, 29*, 575–609.

Fonagy, P., Luyten, P., Moulton-Perkins, A., Lee, Y-W, Warren, F., Howard, S., Ghinai, R. Fearon, P., & Lowyck, B. (2016). Development and Validation of a Self-Report Measure of Mentalizing: The Reflective Functioning Questionnaire. *PLoS One, 11*, 1–28.

Fonagy, P., Steele, H., & Steele, M. (1991). Maternal representations of attachment during pregnancy predict the organization of infant–mother attachment at one year of age. *Child Development, 62*, 891–905.

Fonagy, P., & Target, M. (2007). Playing with reality: IV. A theory of external reality rooted in intersubjectivity. *International Journal of Psychoanalysis, 88*, 917–937.

Fonagy, P., Target, M., & Gergely. G. (2006), Psychoanalytic perspectives on developmental psychopathology. In D. Cicchetti & D. J. Cohen (Eds.), *Developmental psychopathology* (2nd ed., Vol. 1, pp. 701–749). Hoboken, NJ: John Wiley & Sons.

Fosshage, J. (2003). Fundamental pathways to change: Illuminating old and creating new relational experience. *International Forum of Psychoanalysis, 12*, 244–251.

Foucault, M. (1979). *The history of sexuality. Vol. 1: An introduction*. London: Allen Lane.

Foucault, M. (1980). *Power/knowledge: Selected interviews and other writings 1972–1977* (C. Gordon, Ed.). Hemel Hempstead: Harvester Wheatsheaf.

Fraley, R. C., & B. W. Roberts. (2005), Patterns of continuity: A dynamic model for conceptualizing the stability of individual differences in psychological constructs across the life course. *Psychological Review, 112*, 60–74.

Frances, A. (2016). Entrenched reductionisms: The bête noire of psychiatry *History of Psychology, 19*, 57–59.

Frank, J. D., & Frank, J. B. (1993). *Persuasion and healing: A comparative study of psychotherapy* (3rd ed.). Baltimore, MD: Johns Hopkins University Press.

Freud, S. (1905). Bruchstück einer Hysterie-Analyse. *Monatschrift für Psychiatrie und Neurologie, 18*, 285–310, 408–465. English translation: Fragment of an analysis of a case of hysteria. Standard Edition, Vol. 7. London, UK: Hogarth Press.

Freud, S. (1910). The future prospects of psychoanalytic therapy. *Standard Edition, 10*, 87–174. London, UK: Hogarth Press.

Freud, S. (1911). The handling of dream-interpretation in psycho-analysis. *Standard Edition, 12*, 91–96. London, UK: Hogarth Press.

Freud, S. (1912a). Recommendations to physicians practising psycho-analysis. *Standard Edition, 12*, 109–120. London, UK: Hogarth Press.

Freud, S. (1912b). The dynamics of transference. *Standard Edition, 12*, 97–108. London, UK: Hogarth Press.

Freud, S. (1913). On beginning the treatment. *Standard Edition, 12*, 123–144. London, UK: Hogarth Press.

Freud, S. (1914/1963). *The history of the psychoanalytic movement. Standard Edition*, 14, 7–66. London, UK: Hogarth Press.

Freud, S. (1918). From the history on an infantile neurosis. *Standard Edition*, 17, 1–122. London, UK: Hogarth Press.

Freud, S. (1919), Lines of advance in psycho-analytic therapy. *Standard Edition*, 17, 157–168. London, UK: Hogarth Press, 1955.

Freud, S. (1933). New introductory lectures on psycho-analysis. *Standard Edition*, 22, 5–182. London, UK: Hogarth Press.

Freud, S. (1933). *The question of a Weltanschauung. Standard Edition*, 22, 158–182. London, UK: Hogarth Press.

Freud, S. (1937). *Analysis terminable and interminable. Standard Edition*, 23. London, UK: Hogarth Press.

Frijda, N. H. (1986). *The emotions*. New York, NY: Cambridge University Press.

Frith, U. (2008). *Autism. A very short introduction*. London: Oxford University Press.

Gabbard, G. O. (2007). 'Bound in a nutshell': Thoughts on complexity, reductionism, and 'infinite space'. *International Journal of Psychoanalysis*, 88(3), 559–574.

Gabbard, G. O., & Westen, D. (2003). Rethinking therapeutic action. *International Journal of Psychoanalysis*, 84, 823–841.

Gadamer, H. (1975). *Truth & method*. New York, NY: Crossroad.

Gazzaniga, M. (2015). *Tales from both sides of the brain: A life in neuroscience*. New York: Harper Collins Publishers.

Gazzaniga, M. (2018). *Psychological science*. New York: Norton.

Geller, S. M., & Greenberg, L. S. (2012). *Therapeutic presence: A mindful approach to effective therapy*. Washington, DC: American Psychological Association.

Gelo, O. C., & Salvatore, S. (2016). A dynamic systems approach to psychotherapy: A meta-theoretical framework for explaining psychotherapy change processes. *Journal of Counseling Psychology*, 63, 379–395.

Gelso, C. J. (2009a). The real relationship in a postmodern world: Theoretical and empirical explorations. *Psychotherapy Research*, 19, 253–264.

Gelso, C. J. (2009b). The time has come: The real relationship in psychotherapy research. *Psychotherapy Research*, 19, 278–282.

Gelso, C.J., Kivlighan, D.M., & Markin, R.D. (2018). The real relationship and its role in psychotherapy outcome: A meta-analysis. *Psychotherapy*, 55, 434–444.

Gendlin, E. T. (1996). *Focusing oriented psychotherapy*. New York: The Guilford Press.

Gentile, J. (2017). Tugging at the Umbilical Cord: Birtherism, Nativism, and the Plotline of Trump's Delivery. *Contemporary Psychoanalysis*, 53, 489–504.

Germer, C., & Neff, K. (2019). *Teaching the mindful self-compassion program: A guide for professionals*. London: The Guilford Press.

Gerson, S. (2004). The relational unconscious: A core element of intersubjectivity, thirdness, and clinical process. *Psychoanalytic Quarterly*, 73, 63–98.

Gerson, S. (2009). When the third is dead: Memory, mourning and witnessing in the aftermath of the Holocaust. *International Journal of Psychoanalysis*, 90, 1341–1357.

Gentile, J. (2007). Wrestling with matter: Origins of intersubjectivity. *Psychoanalytic Quarterly*, 76. 547–582.

Ghent, E. (1989). Credo: The dialectics of one-person and two-person psychologies. *Contemporary Psychoanalysis*, 25, 169–211.

Ghent, E. (1990). Masochism, submission, surrender. *Contemporary Psychoanalysis, 26,* 169–211.

Giddens, A. (1991). *Modernity and self-identity: Self and society in the late modern age.* Stanford University Press.

Gilbert, P. (2005). *Compassion: conceptualisations, research and use in psychotherapy* London: Routledge.

Gill, M. M. (1954). Psychoanalysis and exploratory psychotherapy. *Journal of the American Psychoanalytic Association, 2,* 771–797.

Gill, M. M. (1984). Psychoanalysis and psychotherapy: A revision. *International Review of Psycho-Analysis, 11,* 161–179.

Glas, G. (2019). *Person-centered care in psychiatry.* London: Routledge.

Glover, E. (1954). The indications for psychoanalysis. *Journal of Mental Science, 100,* 393–401.

Goldberg, S. B., Hoyt, W. T., Nissen-Lie, H. A., Nielsen, S. L., & Wampold, B. E. (2018). Unpacking the therapist effect: Impact of treatment length differs for high- and low-performing therapists. *Psychotherapy Research, 28,* 532–544.

Goldberg, S. B., Rousmaniere, T., Miller, S. D., Whipple, J., Nielsen, S. L., Hoyt, W. T., & Wampold, B. E. (2016). Do psychotherapists improve with time and experience? A longitudinal analysis of outcomes in a clinical setting. *Journal of Counseling Psychology, 63,* 1–11.

Goldfried, M. (2010). Building a two-way bridge between practice and research. *Clinical Psychologist: Newsletter, Div. 12, Amer. Psychol. Assn., 63*(1), 1–3.

Govrin, A. (2016). *Conservative and radical perspectives on psychoanalytic knowledge.* London: Routledge.

Grant, R. W. (1997). *Hypocrisy and integrity. Machiavelli, Rousseau, and the ethics of politics.* Chicago: University of Chicago Press.

Green, A. (1986). *On private madness.* London: Hogarth.

Green A (1995). Has sexuality anything to do with psychoanalysis? *International Journal of Psychoanalysis, 76,* 871–883.

Greenberg, J. (2001). The analyst's participation: A new look. *Journal of the American Psychoanalytic Association, 49,* 359–381.

Greenberg, L.S. (2008). Emotion and cognition in psychotherapy: The transforming power of affect. *Canadian Psychology, 49,* 49–59.

Greenberg, L. S. (2011). *Emotion-focused therapy. Theories of psychotherapy series.* Washington, DC: American Psychological Association.

Greenberg, J., & Mitchell, S. A. (1983). *Objects relations in psychoanalytic theory.* Cambridge, MA: Harvard University Press.

Greenberg, L. S., & Pascual-Leone, A. (2006). Emotion in psychotherapy: A practice-friendly research review. *Journal of Clinical Psychology, 62*(5), 611–630.

Greenson, R. R. (1965). The working alliance and the transference neurosis. *Psychoanalytic Quarterly, 34,* 155–179.

Greenson, R. R. (1967). *The technique and practice of psychoanalysis.* New York: International Universities Press.

Grepmair, L., Mitterlehner, F., Loew, T., Bachler, E., Rother, W., & Nickel, M. (2007). Promoting mindfulness in psychotherapists in training influences the treatment results of their patients: A randomized, double-blind, controlled study. *Pychotherapy and Psychosomatics, 76,* 332–338.

Groh, A. M., Narayan, A. J., Bakermans-Kranenburg, M. J., Roisman, G. I., Vaughn, B. E., Fearon, R. M. P., & van IJzendoorn, M. H. (2017). Attachment and temperament in the early life course: A meta-analytic review. *Child Development, 88*, 770–795.

Grossmark, R. (2012). The flow of enactive engagement. *Contemporary Psychoanalysis, 48*, 287–300.

Gunderson, J. (2007). Alternative perspectives on psychodynamic psychotherapy of borderline personality disorder: The case of "Ellen". *American Journal of Psychiatry, 164*, 1333–1339.

Gunderson, J. G., Bateman, A., & Kernberg, O. (2007). Alternative perspectives on psychodynamic psychotherapy of borderline personality disorder: The case of "Ellen". *American Journal of Psychiatry, 164*, 1333–1339.

Ham, J., & Tronick, E. (2009). Relational psychophysiology: Lessons from mother-infant physiology research on dyadically expanded states of consciousness. *Psychotherapy Research, 19*, 619– 632.

Hannan, C., Lambert, M. J., Harmon, C., Nielsen, S. L., Smart, D. W., Shimokawa, K., & Sutton, S. W. (2005). A lab test and algorithms for identifying clients at risk for treatment failure. *Journal of Clinical Psychology, 61(2)*, 155–163.

Hare B., & Woods, V. (2020). Survival of the friendliest: Natural selection for hypersocial traits enabled Earth's apex species to best Neandertals and other competitors. *Scientific American, 323*, 58–63.

Harrington, A. (2019). *Mind fixers: Psychiatry's troubled search for the biology of mental illness*. New York: W. W. Norton & Company.

Harris, T., Lepper, G., Cheetham, B., Crowther, C., King, D & Ryde, J. (2020). Bridging the gap between clinical practice and research. Part I: Findings of a pilot study on Daniel Stern's 'moments of meeting' from the UKCP's Practitioner Research Network. *British Journal of Psychotherapy, 36*, 180–199.

Hatcher, R. L., & Barends, A. W. (2006). How a return to theory could help alliance research. *Psychotherapy: Theory, Research, & Practice, 43*, 292–299.

Hatfield, D., McCullough, L., Frantz, S. H., & Krieger, K. (2010). Do we know when our clients get worse? An investigation of therapists' ability to detect negative client change. *Clinical Psychology & Psychotherapy, 17(1)*, 25–32.

Hayes, J. A., Gelso, C. J., Goldberg, S., & Kivlighan, D. M. (2018). Countertransference management and effective psychotherapy: Meta-analytic findings. *Psychotherapy, 55*, 496–507.

Hayes, J. A., Gelso, C. J., & Hummel, A. M. (2011). Managing countertransference. *Psychotherapy, 48*, 88–97.

Hayes, A. M., Laurenceau, J.-P., & Cardaciotto, L. (2008). Methods for capturing the process of change. In A. M. Nezu, & C Maguth (Eds.), *Evidence-based outcome research: A practical guide to conducting randomized controlled trials for psychosocial interventions*. London: Oxford University Press.

Hayes, S. C., Strosahl, K. D., & Wilson, K. G. (2012). *Acceptance and commitment therapy: The process and practice of mindful change* (2nd ed.). New York: Guilford Press.

Hayes, J. A., & Vinca, M. (2017). Therapist presence, absence, and extraordinary presence. In L. Castonguay & C. Hill (Eds.), *How and why are some therapists better than others? Understanding therapist effects*. American Psychological Association.

Haynes, S. N., & O'Brien, W. H. (1990). Functional analysis in behavior therapy. *Clinical Psychology Review, 10*, 649–668.

Heath, C. (1992). The delivery and reception of diagnosis and assessment in the general practice consultation. In P. Drew & J. Heritage (Eds.), *Talk at work.* Cambridge: Cambridge University Press.

Hegel, G. W. F. (1977). *Phenomenology of spirit.* Oxford: Oxford University Press. Originally published in 1807; trans. A. V. Miller.

Heidegger, M. (1927). Sein und Zeit.

Heimann, P. (1950). On countertransference. *International Journal of Psycho-Analysis, 31,* 81–84.

Heinonen, E., & Nissen-Lie, H. A. (2019). The professional and personal characteristics of effective psychotherapists: A systematic review. *Psychotherapy Research, 30,* 417–432.

Heritage, J., & Clayman, S. (2010). *Talk in action: Interactions, identities, and institutions.* Chichester: Wiley-Blackwell.

Hill, C. E. (2004). Immediacy. In C. Hill (Ed.), *Helping skills: Facilitating exploration, insight, and action* (2nd ed., pp. 283–297). Washington, DC: American Psychological Association.

Hill, C. (2010). Qualitative studies of negative experiences in psychotherapy. In J. C. Muran & J. P. Barber (Eds.), *The therapeutic alliance: An evidence-based guide to practice.* New York: The Guilford Press.

Hill, C. E., & Knox, S. (2002). Self-disclosure. *Psychotherapy, 38,* 412–416.

Hill, C. E., Knox, S., & Pinto-Coelho, K. G. (2018). Therapist self-disclosure and immediacy: A qualitative meta-analysis. *Psychotherapy, 55,* 445–460.

Hill, C. E., Thompson, B. J., Cogar, M. C., & Denman, D. W. (1993). Beneath the surface of long-term therapy: Therapist and client report of their own and each other's covert processes. *Journal of Counseling Psychology, 40,* 278 –287.

Hoffman, I. Z. (1983). The patient as interpreter of the analyst's experience. *Contemporary Psychoanalysis, 19,* 389–422.

Hoffman, I. Z. (1994). Dialectical thinking and therapeutic action in the psychoanalytic process. *Psychoanalytic Quarterly, 63,* 187–218.

Hoffman, I. Z. (1996), The intimate and ironic authority of the analyst. *Psychoanalytic. Quarterly, 65,* 102–136.

Hoffman, I. Z. (1998). *Ritual and spontaneity in the psychoanalytic process: A dialectical-constructivist view.* Hillsdale, NJ: The Analytic Press.

Hoffman, I. Z. (2006). The myths of free association and the potentials of the analytic relationship. *International Journal of Psychoanalysis, 87,* 43–61.

Hoffman, I.Z. (2009a) Doublethinking our way to 'scientific' legitimacy: The dessication of human experience. *Journal of the American Psychoanalytic Association, 57,* 1043–1069.

Hoffman, I. Z. (2009b). Therapeutic passion in the countertransference. *Psychoanalytic Dialogues, 19,* 617–637.

Hoffman, I. Z. (2016). The risks of therapist passivity and the potentials of constructivist influence. *Psychoanalytic Dialogues, 26,* 91–97.

Hofmann, S. G., Asnaani, A., Vonk, I. J., Sawyer, A. T., & Fang, A. (2012). The efficacy of cognitive behavioral therapy: A review of meta-analyses. *Cognitive Therapy & Research, 36,* 427–440.

Hofmann, S. G., & Hayes, S. C. (2019). The future of intervention science: Process-based therapy. *Clinical Psychological Science*, 7, 37–50.

Hoglend, P., Amlo, S., Marble, A., Bogwald, K.-P., Sorbye, O., Sjaastad, M. C., et al. (2006). Analysis of the patient-therapist relationship in dynamic psychotherapy: An experimental study of transference interpretations. *American Journal of Psychiatry*, *163*, 1739–1746.

Hoglend, P., Bogwald, K.-P., Amlo, S., Marble, A., Ulberg, R., Sjaastad, M. C., et al. (2008). Transference interpretations in dynamic psychotherapy: Do they really yield sustained effects? *American Journal of Psychiatry*, *165*, 763–771.

Høglend, P., & Gabbard, G. O. (2012). When is transference work useful in psychodynamic psychotherapy? A review of empirical research. In R. A. Levy, J. S. Ablon, H. Kächele (Eds.), *Psychodynamic psychotherapy research: Evidence-based practice and practice-based evidence*. Totowa, NJ: Humana Press – Springer.

Høglend, P., & Hagtvet, K. (2019). Change mechanisms in psychotherapy: Both improved insight and improved affective awareness are necessary. *Journal of Consulting and Clinical Psychology*, *87*, 332–344.

Holmes, J., & Slade, A. (2018). *Attachment in Therapeutic Practice*. London: Sage.

Holmqvist, R. (2000). Staff feelings and patient diagnosis. *Canadian Journal of Psychiatry*, *45* (2), 349–356.

Holmqvist, R. (2001). Patterns of consistency and deviation in therapists' countertransference feelings. *Journal of Psychotherapy Practice & Research*, *10*, 104–116.

Holmqvist, R., & Andersen, K. (2003). Therapists "reactions to treatment of survivors of political torture. *Professional Psychology: Research and Practice*, 34, 294–300.

Holmqvist, R., & Armelius, K. (2004). Associations between psychiatric patients' self-image, staff feelings towards them, and treatment outcome. *Psychiatry Research*, *128*, 89–102.

Holmqvist, R., Hansjons-Gustafsson, U., & Gustafsson, J. (2002). Patients' relationship episodes and therapists' feelings. *Psychology and Psychotherapy: Theory, Research and Practice*, 75, 393–409.

Holsti, O. (1969). *Content analysis for the social sciences and humanities*. Reading, MA: Addison-Wesley.

Horvath, A. O. (2018). Research on the alliance: Knowledge in search of a theory. *Psychotherapy Research*, *28*, 499–516.

Houellebecq, M. (2002). *Platform*. London: Heineman.

Howell, E. (2011). *Understanding and treating dissociative identity disorder: A relational approach*. New York, NY: Routledge/Taylor & Francis Group.

Insel, T., Cuthbert, B., Carvey, M., Heinssen, R. Pine, D. S., Quinn, K., Sanislow, C., & Wang, P. (2010). Research Domain Criteria (RDoC): Toward a new classification framework for research on mental disorders. *American Journal of Psychiatry*, *167*, 748–751.

Ivey, G. (2015). The mindfulness status of psychoanalytic psychotherapy. *Psychoanalytic Psychotherapy*, *29*, 382–398.

Jacobs, T. (1991), The interplay of enactments: Their role in the analytic process. In T. Jacobs (Ed.), *The use of the self*. Madison, CT: International Universities Press.

Jacoby, R. (1986). *The repression of psychoanalysis: Otto Fenichel and the political Freudians*. Chicago: University of Chicago Press.

Jaycox, L. H., Foa, E.B., & Morral, A. R. (1998). Influence of emotional engagement and habituation on exposure therapy for PTSD. *Journal of Consulting and Clinical Psychology, 66 (1)*, 185–192.

Jimenez, J. P. (2009). Grasping psychoanalysts' practice in its own merits. *The International Journal of Psychoanalysis 90*, 231–248.

Johansson, P., Hoglend, P., Ulberg, R., Amlo, S., Marble, A., Bogwald, K., Sörbye, O., Sjaastad, M.C., Heyerdahl, O. (2010). The mediating role of insight for long-term improvements in psychodynamic therapy. *Journal of Consulting & Clinical Psychology 78*:438–448.

Johns, R. G., Barkham, M., Kellett, S., & Saxon, D. (2019). A systematic review of therapist effects: A critical narrative update and refinement to Baldwin and Imel's (2013) review. *Clinical Psychology Review, 67*, 78–93.

Johnstone, L., & Boyle, M. with Cromby, J., Dillon, J., Harper, D., Kinderman, P., Longden, E., Pilgrim, D., & Read, J. (2018). *The power threat meaning framework: Towards the identification of patterns in emotional distress, unusual experiences and troubled or troubling behaviour, as an alternative to functional psychiatric diagnosis.* Leicester: British Psychological Society.

Jones. E. (1955). *The life and work of Sigmund Freud.* New York: Basic Books.

Jurist, E. (2018). *Minding emotions. Cultivating mentalization in psychotherapy.* London: Guilford.

Kahn, E. (1985). Heinz Kohut and Carl Rogers: A timely comparison. American Psychologist, *40*(8), 893–904.

Kahn, E. (1989). Carl Rogers and Heinz Kohut: Toward a constructive collaboration. *Psychotherapy, 26*, 555–563.

Kahn, E., & Rachman, A. W. (2000). Carl Rogers and Heinz Kohut: A historical perspective. *Psychoanalytic Psychology, 17*, 294–312.

Kahneman, D. (2011). *Thinking, fast and slow.* New York: MacMillan.

Kanai R., Bahrami, B., Duchaine, B., Janik, A., Banissy, M. J., & Rees, G. (2012). Brain structure links loneliness to social perception. *Current Biology, 22*, 1975–1979.

Kashdan, T. B., Barrett, L. F., & McKnight, P. E. (2015). Unpacking emotion differentiation; transforming unpleasant experience by perceiving distinctions in negativity. *Current Directions in Psychological Science, 24(1)*, 10–16.

Kazdin, A. E. (2005). Treatment outcomes, common factors, and continued neglect of mechanisms of change. *Clinical Psychology: Science and Practice, 12*, 184–188.

Kazdin, A. E. (2009). Understanding how and why psychotherapy leads to change. *Psychotherapy Research, 19*, 418–428.

Kernberg, O. F. (2001). Recent developments in the technical approaches of English-language psychoanalytic schools. *Psychoanalytic Quarterly, 70*, 519–547.

Kernberg, O. F. (2002). Psychoanalytic contributions to psychiatry. *Arch Gen Psychiatry, 59*, 497–498.

Keselman, H., Osvaldsson Cromdal, K., Kullgard, N., & Holmqvist, R. (2018). Responding to mentalization invitations in psychotherapy sessions – a conversation analysis approach. *Psychotherapy Research, 28*, 654–666.

Kiesler, D. J. (1966). Some myths of psychotherapy research and the search for a paradigm. *Psychological Bulletin, 65*, 110–136.

Kiesler, D. J. (1986). Interpersonal methods of diagnosis and treatment. In J. O. Cavenar (Ed.), *Psychiatry* (Vol. 1). Philadelphia: Lippincott.

Kluft, R. P. (1999). An overview of the psychotherapy of dissociative identity disorder. *American Journal of Psychotherapy*, *53*, 289–319.

Knoblauch, S. H. (2000). *The musical edge of therapeutic dialogue*. Analytic Press.

Knoblauch, S. (2018). Core competency five: Patterning and linking. In R. E. Barsness (Ed.), *Core competencies of relational psychoanalysis: A guide to practice, study, and research*. London: Routledge.

Kochiyama, T., Ogihara, N., Tanabe, H. C., Kondo O, Amano H, Hasegawa K, Suzuki H, Ponce de León MS, Zollikofer CPE, Bastir M, Stringer C, Sadato N, Akazawa T.Kochiyama T, et al. (2018). Reconstructing the Neanderthal brain using computational anatomy. *Scientific Reports*, *26*, 6296.

Koelen, J., P. Luyten, E. H. Eurelings-Bontekoe, L. Diguer, R. Vermote, B. Lowyck, & M. Bühring. (2012), The impact of level of personality organization on treatment response: A systematic review. *Psychiatry: Interpersonal and Biological Processes*, 75(4), 355–374.

Kohlenberg, R., & Tsai, M. (1991). *Functional analytic psychotherapy: Creating intense and curative therapeutic relationships*. New York: Plenum Press.

Kohut, H. (1959). Introspection, empathy, and psychoanalysis: An examination of the relationship between mode of observation and theory. *Journal of the American Psychoanalytic Association*, *7*, 459–483

Kohut, H. (1971). *The analysis of the self*. New York: International Universities Press.

Kohut, H. (1984). In A. Goldberg & P. Stepansky (Eds.), *How does analysis cure?* Chicago: University of Chicago Press.

Krall, H. (1992). *The subtenant/To outwit God*. Chicago: Northwestern University Press.

Kuutmann, K., & Hilsenroth, M. J. (2012). Exploring in-session focus on the patient-therapist relationship: Patient characteristics, process and outcome. *Clinical Psychology and Psychotherapy*, *19*, 187–202.

Kvaale, E. P., Haslam, N., & Gottdiener, W. H. (2013). The 'side effects' of medicalization: A meta-analytic review of how biogenetic explanations affect stigma. *Clinical Psychology Review*, *33*, 782–794.

Lakoff, G. (1973). Hedges: A study of meaning criteria and the logic of fuzzy concepts. *Journal of Philosophical Logic*, *2*, 458–508.

Lambert, M. J. (2013). The efficacy and effectiveness of psychotherapy. In M. J. Lambert (Ed.), *Bergin & Garfield's handbook of psychotherapy and behavior change* (6th ed.). New York, NY: Wiley.

Lambert, M. J., Whipple, J. L., & Kleinstäuber, M. (2018). Collecting and delivering progress feedback: A meta-analysis of routine outcome monitoring. *Psychotherapy*, 55(4), 520–537.

Langs, R. J. (1995). *The psychotherapeutic conspiracy*. New York: Jason Aronson.

Laska, K. M., Gurman, A. S., & Wampold, B. E. (2014). Expanding the lens of evidence-based practice in psychotherapy: A common factors perspective. *Psychotherapy*, *51*, 467–481.

Layton, L. (2014). Grandiosity, neoliberalism and neoconservatism. *Psychoanalytic Inquiry*, *34*, 463–474.

Layton, L. (2018). Relational theory in socio-historical context. In L. Aron, S. Grand, & J. Slochower (Eds.), *De-Idealizing Relational Theory*. London: Routledge.

Layton, L., Hollander, N. C., & Gutwill, S. (2006). *Psychoanalysis, class, and politics. Encounters in the clinical setting*. London: Routledge.

Lear, J. (2003). *Therapeutic action: An earnest plea for irony*. London: Karnac.

Leichsenring, F., Kruse, J., & Rabung, S. (2015). Efficacy of psychodynamic psychotherapy in specific mental disorders: An update. In P. Luyten, L. C. Mayes, P. Fonagy, M. Target, & S. Blatt (Eds.), *Handbook of psychodynamic approaches to psychopathology*. London: The Guilford Press.

Leichsenring, F., Luyten, P., Hilsenroth, M. J., Abbass, A., Barber, J. P.; Keefe, J. R., Leweke, F., Rabung, S., & Steinert, C. (2015). Psychodynamic therapy meets evidence-based medicine: A systematic review using updated criteria. *The Lancet Psychiatry, 2*, 648–660.

Levenson, H. (2017). *Brief dynamic therapy*. New York: American Psychological Association.

Levenson, E. A., & Feiner, A. H. (Eds.). (1991). *The purloined self: Interpersonal perspectives in psychoanalysis*. New York: Contemporary Psychoanalysis Books.

Levinas, E. (1972). *Humanisme de l'autre Home*. Montpellier: Fata Morgana.

Lilliengren, P., Johansson, R., Lindqvist, K., Mechler, J., & Andersson, G. (2016). Efficacy of experiential dynamic therapy for psychiatric conditions: A meta-analysis of randomized controlled trials. *Psychotherapy, 53*, 90–104.

Linehan, M. M. 2015). *DBT Skills Training Manual*. New York: Guilford.

Lingiardi, V., Holmqvist, R., & Safran, J. D. (2016). Relational turn and psychotherapy research. *Contemporary Psychoanalysis, 52*, 275–312, 2016.

Loewald, H. (1960). The therapeutic action of psychoanalysis. In *Papers on psychoanalysis*. New Haven, CT: Yale University Press.

Lomas, T., Medina, J. C.S., Ivtzan, I., Rupprecht, S., Eiroa-Orosa, & Francisco José, A. (2018). Systematic review of the impact of mindfulness on the well-being of healthcare professionals. *Journal of Clinical Psychology, 74*, 319–355.

Lord, S. (2017). *Moments of meeting in psychoanalysis. Interaction and change in the Therapeutic Encounter*. Relational Perspectives Book Series. London: Routledge.

Lorenzo-Luaces, L., & DeRubeis, R. J. (2018). Miles to go before we sleep: Advancing the understanding of psychotherapy by modeling complex processes. *Cognitive Therapy and Research, 42*, 212–217.

Luborsky, L. (1976). Helping alliances in psychotherapy: The groundwork for a study of their relationship to its outcome. In J. L. Claghorn (Ed.), *Successful therapy*. New York: Brunner/Mazel.

Luborsky, L. (1984). *Principles of psychoanalytic psychotherapy: A manual for supportive-expressive treatment*. New York: Basic Books.

Luborsky, L., & Crits-Christoph, P. (1990). *Understanding transference*. New York: Basic Books.

Lunbeck, E. (2014). *The Americanization of narcissism*. Cambridge, MA: Harvard University Press.

Luyten, P. L. (2015). Unholy questions about five central tenets of psychoanalysis that need to be empirically verified. *Psychoanalytic Inquiry, 35*, 5–23.

Luyten, P., & Blatt, S. J. (2012). Psychodynamic treatment of depression. *Psychiatric Clinics of North America, 35*, 111–129.

Luyten, P., L. C. Mayes, M. Target, & P. Fonagy. (2012). Developmental research. In G. O. Gabbard, B. Litowitz, & P. Williams (Eds.), *Textbook of psychoanalysis* (2nd ed.). Washington, DC: American Psychiatric Press.

Lyons-Ruth K. (1999). The two-person unconscious: Intersubjective dialogue, enactive relational representation, and the emergence of new forms of relational organization. *Psychoanalytic Inquiry, 19*, 576–617.

MacDonald, J., & Muran, C. J. (2020). The reactive therapist: The problem of interpersonal reactivity in psychological therapy and the potential for a mindfulness-based program focused on "Mindfulness-in-Relationship" skills for therapists. *Journal of Psychotherapy Integration.* Advance online publication.

MacIntosh, H. B. (2015). Titration of technique: Clinical exploration of the integration of trauma model and relational psychoanalytic approaches to the treatment of dissociative identity disorder. *Psychoanalytic Psychology, 32*, 517–538.

Magnenat, L. (2016). Psychosomatic breast and alexithymic breast: A Bionian psychosomatic perspective. *The International Journal of Psychoanalysis, 97*, 41–63.

McDougall, J. (1993). *Plea for a measure of abnormality.* London: Routledge.

McWilliams, N. (1999). *Psychoanalytic case formulation.* New York: Guilford Press.

McWilliams, N. (2004). *Psychoanalytic psychotherapy: A practitioner's guide.* New York: Guilford Press.

Mahler, S., Pine, M.M., & Bergman, A. (1973). *The Psychological Birth of the Human Infant.* New York: Basic Books.

Mahoney, P. (1996). *Freud's Dora: A Psychoanalytic, Historical and Textual Study.* New Haven, CT: Yale University Press.

Mahoney, P. (2005). Freud's unadored and unadorable: A case history terminable and interminable. *Psychoanalytic Inquiry, 25*, 27–44.

Main, M., Goldwyn, R., & Hesse, E. (2003). Adult attachment classification system version 7.2. Unpublished manuscript, University of California, Berkeley.

Malan, D. H. (1963). *A study of brief psychotherapy.* New York: Plenum Press.

Mander, J., Blanck, P., Neubauer, A. B., Kröger, P., Flückiger, C., Lutz, W., & Heidenreich, T. (2019). Mindfulness and progressive muscle relaxation as standardized session introduction in individual therapy: A randomized controlled trial. *Journal of Clinical Psychology, 75*, 21–45.

Mann, J. (1973). *Time-limited psychotherapy.* Cambridge, MA: Harvard University Press.

Mark, D. (2018). Forms of equality in relational psychoanalysis. In L. Aron, S. Grand, & J. Slochower (Eds.), *De-idealizing relational theory. A critique from within.* London: Routledge.

Markowitz, J. C., Milrod, B., Luyten, P., & Holmqvist, R. (2019). Mentalizing in Interpersonal Psychotherapy. *American Journal of Psychotherapy.* Online in advance publication.

Maroda, K. (2002). No place to hide: Affectivity, the unconscious, and the development of relational techniques. *Contemporary Psychoanalysis, 38*, 101–120.

Martin, L. H., Gutman, H., & Hutton, P. H. (1988). *Technologies of the self. A seminar with Michel Foucault.* London: Tavistock.

Mayes, L. C., Patrick Luyten, Sidney J. Blatt, Peter Fonagy, & Mary Target. (2015). Future Perspectives. In P. Luyten, L. C. Mayes, P. Fonagy, M. Target, & S. Blatt (Eds.), *Handbook of psychodynamic approaches to psychopathology.* London: The Guilford Press.

Mayotte-Blum, J., Slavin-Mulford, J., Lehmann, M., Pesale, F., Becker-Matero, N., & Hilsenroth, M. (2012). Therapeutic immediacy across long-term psychodynamic psychotherapy: An evidence-based case study. *Journal of Counseling Psychology*, *59*, 27–40.

McAleavey, A. A., & Castonguay, L. G. (2014). Insight as a common and specific impact of psychotherapy: Therapist-reported exploratory, directive, and common factor interventions. *Psychotherapy*, *51*, 283–294.

McCarthy, P. R., & Betz, N. E. (1978). Differential effects of self-disclosing versus self-involving counselor statements. *Journal of Counseling Psychology*, *25*. 251–256.

McCullough, L., Kuhn, N., Andrews, S., Kaplan, A., Wolf, J., & Hurley, C. L. (2003). *Treating affect phobia. Treating affect phobia: A manual for short-term dynamic psychotherapy*. London: Guilford Press.

McCullough, L., Winston, A., Farber, B. A., Porter, F., Pollack, J., Vingiano, W., Laikin, M., & Trujillo, M. (1991). The relationship of patient-therapist interaction to outcome in brief psychotherapy. *Psychotherapy: Theory, Research, Practice, Training*, *28*, 525–533.

McDonnell, A., McCreadie, M., Mills, R., Deveau, R., Anker, R., & Hayden, J. (2015). The role of physiological arousal in the management of challenging behaviours in individuals with autistic spectrum disorders. *Research in Developmental Disabilities*, *36*, 311–322.

McKay, R. K. (2019). Bread and roses: Empathy and recognition. *Psychoanalytic Dialogues*, *29*, 75–91.

McLaughlin, J. (1991). Clinical and theoretical aspects of enactment. *Journal of the American Psychoanalytic Association*, *39*, 595–614.

Mearns, D., & Cooper, M. (2005). *Working at relational depth in counselling and psychotherapy*. London: Sage.

Merleau-Ponty, M. (1945/1962). *Phenomenology of perception*. New York: Routledge.

Meltzoff, A., & Moore, M. K. (1998). Infant intersubjectivity: Broadening the dialogue to include imitation, identity and intention. In S. Braaten (Ed.), *Intersubjective communication and emotion in early ontogeny*. Cambridge, UK: Cambridge University Press.

Mesquita, B., Boiger, M., & De Leersnyder, J. (2016). The cultural construction of emotions. *Current Opinion in Psychology*, *8*, 31–36.

Messer, S., & McWilliams, N. (2007). Insight in psychodynamic therapy: Theory and assessment. In L. G. Castonguay & C. E. Hill (Eds.), *Insight in psychotherapy*. Washington, DC: American Psychological Association.

Michalak, J., & Holtforth, M. G. (2006). Where do we go from here? The goal perspective in psychotherapy. *Clinical Psychology: Science and Practice*, *13*, 346–365.

Mikulincer, M., Shaver, P. R., & Berant, E. (2013). An attachment perspective on therapeutic processes and outcomes. *Journal of Personality*, *81*, 606–616.

Miller-Bottome, M., Talia, A., Safran, J. D., Muran, J. C. (2018). Resolving alliance ruptures from an attachment-informed perspective. *Psychoanalytic Psychology*, *35*, 175–183.

Milrod B, Chambless DL, Gallop R, Busch FN, Schwalberg M, McCarthy KS, et al. (2016). Psychotherapies for panic disorder: A tale of two sites. *Journal of Clinical Psychiatry*, *77*, 927–935.

Mitchell, S. A. (1988). *Relational concepts in psychoanalysis*. Cambridge, MA: Harvard University Press.

Mitchell, S. A. (1993). *Hope and dread in psychoanalysis*. New York, NY: Basic Books.

Mitchell, S. A. (1997). *Influence and autonomy in psychoanalysis*. Hillsdale, NJ: The Analytic Press.

Mitchell, S. A. (1998). The analyst's knowledge and authority. *The Psychoanalytic Quarterly, 67*, 1–31.

Mitchell, S. A. (2000). *Relationality: from attachment to intersubjectivity*. New York: Analytic Press.

Mitchell, S.A., & Aron, L. (Eds.). (1999) *Relational Psychoanalysis: The Emergence of a Tradition*. Hillsdale, NJ: Analytic Press.

Möller, C.   (2018). Mentalizing: Competence and process. (Doctoral dissertation). Linköping: Linköping University Electronic Press.

Möller, C. (2020). *Mentalizing in the therapeutic interaction: A relational perspective*. Manuscript.

Muntigl, P., & Horvath, A. O. (2014). "I can see some sadness in your eyes": When experiential therapists notice a client's affectual display. *Research on Language and Social Interaction, 47*, 89–108.

Muntigl, P., & Horvath, A. O. (2014). The therapeutic relationship in action: How therapists and clients co-manage relational disaffiliation. *Psychotherapy Research, 24*, 327–345.

Muran, J. C. (2007). A relational turn on thick description. In J. C. Muran (Ed.), *Dialogues on difference: Diversity studies of the therapeutic relationship*. Washington, DC: American Psychological Association.

Muran, J.C. (2019). Confessions of a New York rupture researcher: An insider's guide and critique. *Psychotherapy Research, 29*, 1–14.

Muran, J. C., & Eubanks, C. F. (2020). *Therapist performance under pressure. Negotiating emotion, difference, and rupture*. Washington, DC.: American Psychological Association.

Muran, J. C., Safran, J. D., Samstag, L. W., & Winston, A. (2005). Evaluating an alliance-focused treatment for personality disorders. *Psychotherapy, 42*, 532–545.

Nijenhuis, E., van der Hart, O., & Steele, K. (2010). Trauma-related structural dissociation of the personality. *Activitas Nervosa Superior, 52*, 1–23.

Nissen-Lie, H. A., Monsen, J. T., Ulleberg, P., & Rønnestad, M. H. (2012). Psychotherapists' self-reports of their interpersonal functioning and difficulties in practice as predictors of patient outcome. *Psychotherapy Research, 23*, 86–104.

Nissen-Lie, H. A., Rønnestad, M. H., Høglend, P. A., Havik, O. E., Solbakken, O. A., Stiles, T. C., & Monsen, J. T. (2017). Love yourself as a person, doubt yourself as a therapist? *Clinical Psychology & Psychotherapy, 24*, 48–60.

Nussbaum, M.   (1994). The therapy of desire: Theory and practice in Hellenistic ethics. Princeton: Princeton University Press.

Oddli, H. W., McLeod, J., Nissen-Lie, H. A., Rønnestad, M. H., & Halvorsen, M. S. (2021). Future orientation in successful therapies: Expanding the concept of goal in the working alliance. *Journal of Clinical Psychology, 77*, 1307–1329.

Oddli, H. W., McLeod, J., Reichelt, S., & Rønnestad, M. H. (2014). Strategies used by experienced therapists to explore client goals in early sessions of psychotherapy. *European Journal of Psychotherapy & Counselling, 16*, 245–266.

Oddli, H. W., & Rønnestad, M. H. (2012). How experienced therapists introduce the technical aspects in the initial alliance formation: Powerful decision makers supporting clients' agency. *Psychotherapy Research*, *22*, 176–193.

Ogden, T. H. (1985). On potential space. *International Journal of Psychoanalysis*, *66*, 129–141.

Ogden T. H. (1988). On the dialectical structure of experience: Some clinical and theoretical implications . *Contemporary Psychoanalysis*, *24*, 17–45.

Ogden, T. H. (1989). *The primitive edge of experience*. New York; Jason Aronson.

Ogden, T. H. (1992). The dialectically constituted/decentred subject of psychoanalysis: I. The Freudian subject. *International Journal of Psychoanalysis*, *73*, 517–526.

Ogden, T. (1994a) The analytic third: Working with intersubjective clinical facts. *International Journal of Psychoanalysis*, *75*, 3–20.

Ogden, T.H. (1994b). *Subjects of Analysis*. Northvale, NJ: Aronson.

Ogden, T. (2001). *Conversations at the frontier of dreaming*. Northvale, NJ: Aronson.

Ogden, T. H. (2004). The analytic third: Implications for psychoanalytic theory and technique. *The Psychoanalytic Quarterly*, *73*, 167–195.

Ogden, T. H. (2018). The feeling of real: On Winnicott's 'Communicating and Not Communicating Leading to a Study of Certain Opposites. *The International Journal of Psychoanalysis*, *99*, 1288–1304.

OPD Task Force. (2008). *Operationalized Psychodynamic Diagnosis OPD-2. Manual of diagnosis and treatment planning*. Göttingen: Hogrefe.

Orange, D. M. (2011). *The suffering stranger: Hermeneutics for everyday clinical practice*. London, UK: Routledge.

Orange, D. M., Atwood, G. E., & Stolorow, R. D. (1997). *Working Intersubjectively*. Hillsdale, NJ: Analytic Press.

O'Shaughnessy, E. (1994). What is a clinical fact? *International Journal of Psychoanalysis*, *75*, 939–947.

Østergård, O. K., Randa, H., & Hougaard, E. (2020). The effect of using the Partners for Change Outcome Management System as feedback tool in psychotherapy – a systematic review and meta-analysis. *Psychotherapy Research*, *30*, 195–212.

Panksepp, J. (2014). Understanding the neurobiology of core positive emotions through animal models: Affective and clinical implications. In J. Gruber & J. T. Moskowitz (Eds), *Positive emotion: Integrating the light sides and dark sides*. Oxford: Oxford University Press.

Pao, P.-N. (1983). Therapeutic empathy and the treatment of schizophrenics. *Psychoanalytic Inquiry*, *3*(1), 145–167.

Patsiopoulos, A.T., & Buchanan, M.J. (2011). The practice of self-compassion in counseling: A narrative inquiry. *Professional Psychology: Research and Practice*, *42*, 301–307.

Pearlman, L. A., & Courtois, C. A. (2005). Clinical applications of the attachment framework: Relational treatment of complex trauma. *Journal of Traumatic Stress*, *18* (5), 449–459.

Peräkylä, A. (2019). Conversation analysis and psychotherapy: Identifying transformative sequences. *Research on Language and Social Interaction*, *52*, 257–280.

Pescosolido, B. A., Martin, J. K., Long, J. S., Medina, T. R., Phelan, J. C., & Link, B. G. (2010). "A disease like any other"? A decade of change in public reactions to schizophrenia, depression, and alcohol dependence. *American Journal of Psychiatry*, *167*, 1321–1330.

Piccirillo, M. L., & Rodebaugh, T. L. (2019). Foundations of idiographic methods in psychology and applications for psychotherapy. *Clinical Psychology Review, 71*, 90–100.

Pine, F. (1988). The four psychologies of psychoanalysis and their place in clinical work. *Journal of the American Psychoanalytic Association, 36*, 571–596.

Piper, W. E., Joyce, A. S., McCallum, M., & Azim, H. F. (1998). Interpretive and supportive forms of psychotherapy and patient personality variables. *Journal of Consulting and Clinical Psychology, 66*, 558–567.

Pizer, S. A. (1998). *Building bridges: The negotiating of paradoxes in psychoanalysis.* Hillsdale, NJ: Analytic Press.

Polanyi, M. (1958). *Personal knowledge. Towards a post-critical philosophy.* Chicago: University of Chicago Press.

Preston, L. (2008). The edge of awareness: Gendlin's contribution to explorations of implicit experience. *International Journal of Psychoanalytic Self Psychology, 3*, 347–369.

Råbu, M., & McLeod, J. (2018). Wisdom in professional knowledge: Why it can be valuable to listen to the voices of senior psychotherapists. *Psychotherapy Research, 28*, 776–792.

Racker, H. (1968). *Transference and Countertransference.* London: Hogarth Press.

Ramseyer, F. (2020) Exploring the evolution of nonverbal synchrony in psychotherapy: The idiographic perspective provides a different picture. *Psychotherapy Research, 30*, 622–634,

Rapaport, David. (1957). Thinking: Vogue and essence. *Contemporary Psychology, 2*, 249–252.

Reading, R. A., Safran, J. D., Origlieri, A., & Muran, J. C., (2019). Investigating therapist reflective functioning, therapeutic process, and outcome. *Psychoanalytic Psychology, 36*, 115–121.

Redmond, B. (2006). *Reflection in action.* Farnham: Ashgate.

Reese, R. J., Toland, M. D., & Hopkins, N. B. (2011). Replicating and extending the good enough level model of change: Considering session frequency. *Psychotherapy Research, 21*, 608–619.

Reich, A. (1951). On countertransference. *International Journal of Psychoanalysis, 32*, 25–31.

Reik, T. (1949). *Listening with the third ear.* New York: Farrar, Straus.

Renik, O. (1993). Analytic interaction: Conceptualizing technique in light of the analyst's irreducible subjectivity. *Psychoanalytic Quarterly, 62*, 553–571.

Renik, O. (1998). The analyst's subjectivity and the analyst's objectivity. *International Journal of Psychoanalysis, 79*:487–497.

Renik, O. (2007). Intersubjectivity, therapeutic action, and analytic technique. *The Psychoanalytic Quarterly, 76*(Suppl. 1), 1547–1562.

Rhodes, R. H., Hill, C. E., Thompson, B. J., & Elliot, R. (1994). Client retrospective recall of resolved and unresolved misunderstanding events. *Journal of Counseling Psychology, 41*(4), 473–483.

Rickman, J. (1957). *Selected contributions to psychoanalysis.* Oxford, UK: Basic Books.

Ringstrom, P. A. (2001). Cultivating the improvisational in psychoanalytic treatment. *Psychoanalytic Dialogues, 11*, 727–754.

Ringstrom, P. A. (2007).Scenes that write themselves: Improvisational moments in relational psychoanalysis. Psychoanalytic Dialogues, 17, 69–99

Rizzolatti, G., Fadiga, L., Gallese, V., & Fogassi, L. (1996). Premotor cortex and the recognition of motor actions. *Cognitive Brain Research, 3*, 131–141.

Roazen, P. (1995). *How Freud worked: First-hand accounts of patients*. Northvale, NJ: Jason Aronson.

Rogers, C. R. (1957). The necessary and sufficient conditions of therapeutic personality change. *Journal of Consulting Psychology, 21*, 95–103.

Rønnestad, M. H., & Skovholt, T. M. (2013). *The developing practitioner: Growth and stagnation of therapists and counselors*. New York & London: Routledge.

Rosen, M. (2012). *Dignity: Its history and meaning*. Cambridge, MA: Harvard University Press.

Rosenfeld, H. (1987). *Impasse and interpretation: Therapeutic and anti-therapeutic factors in the psychoanalytic treatment of psychotic, borderline, and neurotic patients*. London: Routledge.

Rosenzweig, S. (1936). Some implicit common factors in diverse methods of psychotherapy. *American Journal of Orthopsychiatry, 6*, 412–415.

Rousmaniere, T. (2016). *Deliberate practice for psychotherapists: A guide to improving clinical effectiveness*. New York: Routledge.

Roustang, F. (1976). *Dire mastery*. Baltimore, MD: Johns Hopkins Press.

Rudden, M., Milrod, B., Target, M., Ackerman, S., & Graf, E. (2006). Reflective functioning in panic disorder patients: A pilot study. *Journal of the American Psychoanalytic Association, 54*, 1339–1343.

Russell, P. (1998). Trauma and the cognitive function of affects. In J. Teicholz & D. Kriegman (Eds.), *Trauma, repetition, and affect regulation: The work of Paul Russell*. New York: Other Press.

Ryle, G. (1949). *The concept of the mind*. Chicago: University of Chicago Press.

Safran, J. D. (1999). Faith, despair, will, and the paradox of acceptance. *Contemporary Psychoanalysis, 35*, 5–23.

Safran, J. D. (2002). Brief relational psychoanalytic treatment. *Psychoanalytic Dialogues, 12*, 171–195.

Safran, J.D. (2012). *Psychoanalysis and psychoanalytic theories*. Washington, DC: American Psychological Association.

Safran, J. D. (2016). Agency, surrender, and grace in psychoanalysis. *Psychoanalytic Psychology, 33*, 58–72.

Safran, J. D. (2017). The unbearable lightness of being: Authenticity and the search for the real. *Psychoanalytic Psychology, 34*, 69–77.

Safran, J. D., Abreu, I., Ogilvie, J., & DeMaria, A. (2011). Does psychotherapy research influence the clinical practice of researchers-clinicians? *Clinical Psychology: Science and Practice, 18*, 357–371.

Safran, J. D., & Muran, J. C. (2000). *Negotiating the therapeutic alliance: A relational treatment guide*. New York, NY: Guilford Press.

Safran, J. D., Muran, J. C., & Eubanks-Carter, C. (2011). Repairing alliance ruptures. *Psychotherapy, 48*, 80–87.

Safran, J. D., & Reading, R. (2008). Mindfulness, metacommunication, and affect regulation in psychoanalytic treatment. In S. F. Hick & T. Bien (Eds.), *Mindfulness and the therapeutic relationship* (pp. 122–140). New York, NY: The Guilford Press.

Salberg, J. (2019). Old objects die hard: Generational ruptures. *Psychoanalytic Dialogues, 29*, 637–652.

Sandberg, J., Gustafsson, S., & Holmqvist, R. (2017). Interpersonally traumatised patients' view of significant and corrective experiences in the psychotherapeutic relationship. *European Journal of Psychotherapy & Counselling, 19*, 175–199,

Sandell, R., Blomberg, J., Lazar, A., Carlsson, J., Broberg, J., & Schubert, J. (2000). Varieties of long-term outcome among patients in psychoanalysis and long-term psychotherapy: A review of findings in the Stockholm Outcome of Psychoanalysis and Psychotherapy Project (STOPPP). *International Journal of Psychoanalysis, 81*, 921–942.

Sandell, R., & Wilczek, A. (2016). Another way to think about psychological change. *European Journal of Psychotherapy and Counselling, 18*, 228–251.

Sander, L. (1977). The regulation of exchange in the infant–caretaker system and some aspects of the context-content relationship. In M. Lewis & L. Rosenblum (Eds.), *Interaction, conversation, and the development of language*. New York: Wiley (pp. 133–156).

Sander, L. (1992). Letter to the Editor. Discussion of Evelyne Schwaber's "Countertransference: The analyst's retreat from the patient's vantage point." *International Journal of. Psychoanalysis, 73*, 582–584.

Sander, L. (2008). In G. Amadei & I. Bianchi (Eds.), *Living systems, evolving consciousness, and the emerging person: A selection of papers from the life work of Louis Sander*. New York, NY: Analytic Press.

Sandler, J., Dare, C., & Holder, A. (1973). Interpretations, other interventions and insight. In J. Sandler (Ed.), *The patient and the analyst: The basis of the psycho-analytic process* (pp. 104–120). New York, NY: Basic Books.

Sandler, J., & Sandler, A.-M. (1994). The past unconscious and the present un-conscious: A contribution to a technical frame of reference. *The Psychoanalytic Study of the Child, 49*, 278–292.

Santorelli, S. (1999). *Heal thy self. Lessons on mindfulness in medicine*. London: Bell Tower.

Sawicki J. (1991). *Disciplining Foucault: Feminism, power and the body*. New York: Routledge.

Saxon, D., & Barkham, M. (2012). Patterns of therapist variability: Therapist effects and the contribution of patient severity and risk. *Journal of Consulting and Clinical Psychology, 80*, 535–546.

Saxon, D., Firth, N., & Barkham, M. (2016). The relationship between therapist effects and therapy delivery factors: Therapy modality, dosage, and non-completion. *Administration and Policy in Mental Health and Mental Health Services Research, 44*, 705–715.

Schacter, D. L. (1996). *Searching for memory*. New York, NY: Basic Books.

Schafer, R. (1983). *The analytic attitude*. New York: Basic Books.

Schore A. N. (2003). *Affect dysregulation and disorders of the self*. New York, NY: Norton.

Schore, A. (2012). *The science of the art of psychotherapy*. New York: W.W. Norton.

Schore, J. R., & Schore, A. N. (2008). Modern attachment theory: The central role of affect regulation in development and treatment. *Clinical Social Work Journal, 36*(1), 9–20.

Schön, D. (1983). *The reflective practitioner: how professionals think in action.* Cambridge: Cambridge University Press.

Searles, H. F. (1975). The patient as therapist to his analyst. In P. Giovacchini (Ed.), *Tactics and techniques in psychoanalytic theory.* New York: Jason Aronson, Inc.

Seikkula, J. (2011). Becoming dialogical: Psychotherapy or a way of life? *The Australian and New Zealand Journal of Family Therapy, 32*, 179–193.

Seligman, S. (2005). Dynamic systems theories as a meta-framework for psychoanalysis. *Psychoanalytic Dialogues, 15*, 285–319.

Seligman, S. (2014). Paying attention and feeling puzzled: The analytic mindset as an agent of therapeutic change. *Psychoanalytic Dialogues, 24*, 648–662.

Seligman, S. (2018). Inaction and puzzlement as interaction. Keeping attention in mind. In L. Aron, S. Grand, & J. Slochower (Eds.), *De-idealizing relational theory. A critique from within.* London. Routledge.

Seligman, S. (2019). Louis Sander and contemporary psychoanalysis: Nonlinear dynamic systems, developmental research, clinical process and the search for core principles. *Psychoanalytic Inquiry, 39*, 15–21.

Shabad, P. (2001). *Despair and the return of hope: Echoes of mourning in psychotherapy.* Northvale, NJ: Aronson.

Shahar, G. (2010), Poetics, pragmatics, schematics, and the psychoanalysis–research dialogue. *Psychoanalytic Psychotherapy, 24*, 315–328.

Shanteau, J. (1992). Competence in experts: The role of task characteristics. *Organizational Behavior and Human Decision Processes, 53*, 252–266.

Shay, J. (1994). *Achilles in Vietnam: Combat trauma and the undoing of character.* New York: Atheneum Publishers/Macmillan Publishing.

Shedler, J. (2010). The efficacy of psychodynamic psychotherapy. *American Psychologist, 65*, 98–109.

Sidnell, J. (2016). A conversation analytic approach to research in early childhood. In A. Farrell, S. Kagan, E. Kay, & M. Tisdall (Eds.), *The Sage handbook of early childhood research.* Newbury Park, CA.

Siegel, D. J. (2001). *The neurobiology of "we": How relationships, the mind, and the brain interact to shape who we are.* Washington, DC: American Psychiatric Publishing.

Sifneos, P. E. (1979). *Short-term dynamic psychotherapy: Evaluation and technique.* New York: Plenum Press.

Silverman, S. (2019). I can't think: Past trauma in present time. *Studies in Gender and Sexuality, 20*, 6–10.

Sirote, A. (2020). The priest and the rabbi meet in a bar: The dialectic between merger and recoil in psychoanalysis. *Psychoanalytic Dialogues, 30*, 336–351.

Slavin, M. O. (1996). Is one self enough? Multiplicity in self organization and the capacity to negotiate relational conflict. Discussion of "How many selves make a person?" by Frank M. Lachmann. *Contemporary Psychoanalysis, 32*, 615–625.

Slavin, J. H. (2007a). Reclaiming desire - Love is not enough. *Psychoanalytic Dialogues, 17*, 811–824.

Slavin, J. H. (2007b). Psychoanalytic training: The absence of thirdness. A review of impossible training: A relational view of psychoanalytic education by Emanuel Berman. *Psychoanalytic Dialogues, 17*, 595–609.

Slavin, M. O. (2019). Does truth matter? Introduction to papers by Jody Davies, Shlomit Gadot, and Donnel Stern. *Psychoanalytic Dialogues, 29,* 159–164.

Slavin, M. O., & Kriegman, D. (1998). Why the analyst needs to change: Toward a theory of conflict, negotiation and mutual influence in the therapeutic process. *Psychoanalytic Dialogues, 8,* 247–284.

Slavin, J., & Pollock, L. (1997). The poisoning of desire: The destruction of agency and the recovery of psychic integrity in sexual abuse. *Contemporary Psychoanalysis, 33,* 573–593.

Slochower, J. (2017). Going too far: Relational heroines and relational excess. *Psychoanalytic Dialogues, 27,* 282–299.

Slochower, J. (2020) Resist this. *Psychoanalytic Dialogues, 30,* 64–72,

Spence, D. P. (1982). *Narrative truth and historical truth. Meaning and interpretation in psychoanalysis.* New York: Norton.

Spence, D. P. (1987). *The Freudian Metaphor. Toward paradigm change in psycho-analysis.* New York: Norton.

Spence, D. P. (1994), The failure to ask the hard questions. In P. F. Talley, H. H. Strupp, & S. F. Butler (Ed.), *Psychotherapy research and practice. Bridging the gap* (pp. 19–38). New York: Basic Books.

Spezzano, C. (1998). Listening and interpreting: How relational analysts kill time between disclosures and enactments. *Psychoanalytic Dialogues, 8,* 237–246.

Sterba, R. (1934). The fate of the ego in analytic therapy. *International Journal of Psychoanalysis, 15,* 117–126.

Stern, D. N. (1971). A microanalysis of mother–infant interaction. *Journal of the American. Academy of. Child Psychiatry, 19,* 501–517.

Stern, D.B. (1983) Unformulated experience: From familiar chaos to creative disorder. *Contemporary Psychoanalysis, 19,* 71–99.

Stern, D. N. (1984). Affect attunement. *Frontiers in Infant Psychiatry, 2,* 3–14.

Stern, D. N. (1985). *The interpersonal world of the infant. A view from psychoanalysis and developmental psychology.* New York: Basic Books.

Stern, D. N. (1985/2000). *The interpersonal world of the infant.* New York: Basic Books.

Stern, D. B. (1994). Empathy is interpretation (and whoever said it wasn't?): Commentary on papers by Hayes, Kiersky and Beebe, and Feiner and Kiersky. *Psychoanalytic Dialogues, 4,* 441–471.

Stern, D. B. (1997). *Unformulated experience.* Hillsdale, NJ: The Analytic Press.

Stern, D. N. (2004). *The present moment in psychotherapy and everyday life.* New York, NY: W.W. Norton and Company.

Stern, D. N. (2004a). *The present moment in psychotherapy and everyday life.* New York: Norton.

Stern, D. N. (2004b). The present moment as a critical moment. *Negotiation Journal, 20,* 365–372.

Stern, D. B. (2010). *Partners in thought: Working with unformulated experience, dissociation, and enactment.* New York, NY: Routledge/Taylor & Francis Group.

Stern, D. B. (2013a). Psychotherapy is an emergent process: In favor of acknowledging hermeneutics and against the privileging of systematic empirical research. *Psychoanalytic Dialogues, 23,* 102–115.

Stern, D. B. (2013b). Field theory in psychoanalysis, part 2: Bionian field theory and contemporary interpersonal/relational psychoanalysis. *Psychoanalytic Dialogues, 23,* 630–645.

Stern, D. B. (2015). The interpersonal field: Its place in american psychoanalysis. *Psychoanalytic Dialogues, 25*, 388–404.

Stern, D. B. (2017). Unformulated experience, dissociation, and *Nachträglichkeit. The Journal of Analytical Psychology, 62*, 501–525.

Stern, D., Sander, L., Nahum, J., Harrison, A., Lyons- Ruth, K., Morgan, Bruschweiler Stern, N., & Tronik, E. (1998). Non-interpretative mechanisms in psychoanalytic therapy. The "something more" than interpretation. *International Journal of Psycho-Analysis, 79*, 903–921.

Stiles, W. B., Honos-Webb, L., & Surko, M. (1998). Responsiveness in psychotherapy. *Clinical Psychology: Science and Practice, 5*, 439–458.

Stolorow, R. D. (1991). The intersubjective context of intrapsychic experience: A decade of psychoanalytic inquiry.*Psychoanalytic Inquiry, 11*, 171–184.

Stolorow, R. D., & Atwood, G. E. (1984). Psychoanalytic phenomenology: Toward a science of human experience. *Psychoanalytic Inquiry, 4*, 87–105

Strachey, J. (1934), The nature of the therapeutic action of psychoanalysis. *International. Journal of Psycho-Analysis, 15*, 17–126.

Strupp, H. H. (1955). An objective comparison of Rogerian and psychoanalytic techniques. *Journal of Consulting Psychology, 19*, 1–7.

Strupp, H. H. (2001). Implications of the empirically supported treatment movement for psychoanalysis. *Psychoanalytic Dialogues, 11*, 605–619.

Sugarman, A. (2006). Mentalization, insightfulness, and therapeutic action: The importance of mental organization. *International Journal of Psychoanalysis, 87*, 965–987

Sullivan, H. S. (1940/1953). *Conceptions of modern psychiatry.* New York, NY: Norton.

Sullivan, H. S. (1953). *The interpersonal theory of psychiatry.* New York: W.W. Norton.

Summers, F. (2013). *The psychoanalytic vision: The experiencing subject, transcendence, and the therapeutic process.* London, UK: Routledge.

Summers, F. (2016). The dialectics of psychoanalytic decision-making. *Psychoanalytic Inquiry, 36*, 538–547.

Summers, R. F., & Barber, J. P. (2011). *Psychodynamic Therapy. A guide to evidence-based practice.* London: Guilford.

Summers, R. J., & Barber, J. P. (2014). *Practicing psychodynamic therapy: A casebook.* New York: Guilford Press.

Svensson, M., Nilsson, T., Perrin, S., Johansson, H., Viborg, G., Falkenström, F., & Sandell, R. (2021). The effect of patients' choice of cognitive behavioural or psychodynamic therapy on outcomes for Panic Disorder: A doubly randomised controlled preference trial. *Psychotherapy & Psychosomatics, 90*, 107–118.

Talia, A., Miller-Bottome, M., & Daniel, S. I. F. (2017). Assessing attachment in psychotherapy: Validation of the patient attachment coding system (PACS). *Clinical Psychology & Psychotherapy, 24*, 149–161.

Tanzilli, A., Muzi, L., Ronningstam, E., & Lingiardi, V. (2017). Countertransference when working with narcissistic personality disorder: An empirical investigation. *Psychotherapy, 54*, 184–194.

Task Force on Promotion and Dissemination of Psychological Procedures, Division of Clinical Psychology of the American Psychological Association. (1995). Training and dissemination of empirically validated psychological treatments: Report and recommendations. *Clinical Psychologist, 48*, 3–23.

Taylor, C. (1989). *Sources of the self: The making of the modern identity*. Cambridge, MA: Harvard University Press.

Taylor, C. (1992). *The ethics of authenticity*. Cambridge, MA: Harvard University Press.

Tomkins, S. S. (1962–1963). *Affect, imagery, consciousness* (Vols. 1 and 2). New York: Springer.

Tomkins, S. S. (1991). *Affect, imagery, consciousness, Volume 3: The negative affects: Anger and fear*. New York: Springer.

Town, J. M., Abbass, A., & Hardy, G. (2011). Short-term psychodynamic psychotherapy for personality disorders: A critical review of randomized controlled trials. *Journal of Personality Disorders, 25*, 723–740.

Tublin, S. (2011). Discipline and freedom in relational technique. *Contemporary Psychoanalysis, 47*, 519–546.

Tublin, S. (2018). Core competency one: Therapeutic intent. In R. E. Barsness, (Ed.), *Core competencies of relational psychoanalysis: A guide to practice, study, and research*. London: Routledge.

Tracey, T. J. G., Wampold, B. E., Lichtenberg, J. W., & Goodyear, R. K. (2014). Expertise in psychotherapy: An elusive goal? *American Psychologist, 69*, 218–229.

Trevarthen, C. (1974), The psychobiology of speech development. *Language and Brain, Developmental Aspects.Neurosciences Research Program Bulletin, 12*, 570–585.

Trevarthen, C. (1977). Descriptive analyses of infant communicative behavior. In H. R. Schaffer (Ed.), *Studies in mother–infant interaction*. London: Academic Press.

Trevarthen, C. (1977).

Trevarthen, C. (1980). Communication and cooperation in early infancy: a description of primary intersubjectivity. In M. Bullowa (Ed.), *Before speech: The beginning of interpersonal communication*. New York: Cambridge University Press.

Tronick, E. (1989). Emotions and emotional communication in infants. *American Psychologist, 44*, 112–119.

Tronick, E.Z. (1998). Dyadically expanded states of consciousness and the process of therapeutic change. *Infant Mental Health Journal, 19*, 290–299.

Tronick, E. Z. (2001). Emotional connections and dyadic consciousness in infant–mother and patient–therapist interactions. *Psychoanalytic. Dialogues, 11*, 187–194.

Tronick, E. Z. (2002), A model of infant mood states and Sanderian affective waves. *Psychoanalytic Dialogues, 12*, 73–99.

Tronick, E. Z. (2003), "Of course all relationships are unique": How co-creative processes generate unique mother–infant and patient–therapist relationships and change other relationships. *Psychoanalytic Inquiry, 23*, 473–491.

Tronick, E. (2007). *The Neurobehavioral and social emotional development of infants and children*. New York: Norton.

Tronick, E., & Beeghly, M. (2011). Infants' meaning-making and the development of mental health problems. *American Psychologist, 66*, 107–119.

Tronick, E., & J. Cohn. (1989), Infant–mother face-to-face interaction: Age and gender differences in coordination and the occurrence of miscoordination. *Child Development*, *60*, 85–92.

Trop, G. S., Burke, M. L., & Trop, J. L. (2002). Thinking dynamically in psychoanalytic theory and practice: A review of intersubjectivity theory. In W. J. Coburn (Ed.), *Transformations in self psychology: Progress in self psychology* (Vol. 20). Milton Park: The Analytic Press/Taylor & Francis Group.

Truijens, F., Zühlke-van Hulzen, L., & Vanheule, S. (2019). To manualize, or not to manualize: Is that still the question? A systematic review of empirical evidence for manual superiority in psychological treatment. *Journal of Clinical Psychology*, *75*, 329–343.

Tsai, M., Kohlenberg, R. J., Kanter, J. W., Kohlenberg, B., Follette, W., & Callaghan, G. (2009). *A guide to functional analytic psychotherapy: Awareness, courage, love and behaviorism*. New York: Springer.

Tschacher, W., Junghan, U. M., & Pfammatter, M. (2012).Towards a taxonomy of common factors in psychotherapy—results of an expert survey. *Clinical Psychology & Psychotherapy*, *21*, 82–96.

Tucker-Drob, E. M., Briley, D. A. (2019). Theoretical concepts in the genetics of personality development. In D. P. McAdams, R. L. Shiner, J. L. Tackett (Eds.), *Handbook of personality development*. London: The Guilford Press.

van Ijzendoorn, M. H. & Bakermans-Kranenburg, M. J. (2008). The distribution of adult attachment representations in clinical groups: A meta-analytic search for patterns of attachment in 105 AAI studies. In H. Steele & M. Steele (Eds.), *Clinical applications of the Adult Attachment Interview*. New York: The Guilford Press.

Vehviläinen, S. (2003). Preparing and delivering interpretations in psychoanalytic interaction. *Text*, *23*, 573–606.

Verhage, M. L., Schuengel, C., Madigan, S., Fearon, R. M. P., Oosterman, M., Cassibba, R., Bakermans-Kranenburg, M. J., & van IJzendoorn, M. H. (2016). Narrowing the transmission gap: A synthesis of three decades of research on intergenerational transmission of attachment. *Psychological Bulletin*, *142*, 337–366.

Viklund, E., Holmqvist, R., & Zetterqvist-Nelson, K. (2010). Client identified important events in the therapeutic relationship: Interactional structures and practices. *Psychotherapy Research*, *20*, 151–164.

Voutilainen, L., & Peräkylä, A. (2016). Interactional practices of psychotherapy. In M. O'Reilly, & J. N. Lester (Eds.), *The Palgrave handbook of adult mental health: Discourse and conversation studies*. London: Palgrave Macmillan/Springer Nature.

Wachtel, P. L. (2008). *Relational theory and the practice of psychotherapy*. New York: Guilford.

Wachtel, P. L. (2014). *Cyclical psychodynamics and the contextual self*. London: Routledge.

Wachtel, P. (2018). Toward integrative a more fully integrative and contextual relational paradigm. In L. Aron, S. Grand & J. Slochower (Eds.), *Decentering relational theory. A comparative critique*. London: Routledge.

Wachtel, P. L., Kruk, J. C., & McKinney, M. K. (2005). Cyclical psychodynamics and integrative relational psychotherapy. In J. C. Norcross & M. R. Goldfried (Eds.), *Handbook of psychotherapy integration*. New York: Oxford Universities Press.

Waelder, R. (1962). Psychoanalysis, scientific method, and philosophy. *Journal of the American Psychoanalytic Association, 10*, 617–637.

Walfish, S., McAlister, B., O'Donnell, P., & Lambert, M. J. (2012). An investigation of self-assessment bias in mental health providers. *Psychological Reports, 110*, 639–644.

Wallin, D. J. (2007). *Attachment in psychotherapy*. New York: Guilford.

Wampold, B. E., & Imel, Z. E. (2015). *The great psychotherapy debate: The evidence for what makes psychotherapy work* (2nd ed.). New York: Routledge.

Wampold, B. E., & Owen, J. (in press). Therapist effects: History, methods, magnitude, and characteristics of effective therapists. In M. Barkham, W. Lutz, & L. G. Castonguay (Eds.), *Bergin and Garfield's handbook of psychotherapy and behavior change* (7th ed.). Wiley.

Watson, J. C., & Wiseman, H. (2021). (Eds). *The responsive psychotherapist: Attuning to clients in the moment*. Washington: American Psychological Association.

Watzke, B., Rüddel, H., Jürgensen, R., Koch, U., Kriston, L., Grothgar, B., & Schulz, H. (2012). Longer term outcome of cognitive-behavioural and psychodynamic psychotherapy in routine mental health care: Randomised controlled trial. *Behaviour Research and Therapy, 50*, 580–587.

Webb, C. A., DeRubeis, R. J., & Barber, J. P. (2010). Therapist adherence/competence and treatment outcome: A meta-analytic review. Journal of Consulting and Clinical Psychology, 78, 200–211.

Weiss, J., Sampson, H., & Mt Zion Psychotherapy Research Group. (1986). *The psychoanalytic process: Theory, clinical observations, and empirical research*. London: Guilford Press.

Weissman, M. M., Markowitz, J. C., & Klerman, G. L. (2018). *The guide to interpersonal psychotherapy. Updated and expanded edition*. Oxford: Oxford University Press.

Westerling, T. W., Drinkwater, R., Laws, H., Stevens, H., Ortega, S., Goodman, D., Beinashowitz, J., & Drill, R. L. (2019). *Psychoanalytic Psychology, 36*, 73–81.

Winnicott, D. W. (1949). Hate in the countertransference. In D. W. Winnicott (Ed.), *Collected Papers: Through Paediatrics to Psycho-Analysis*. London: Tavistock, 1958.

Winnicott , D. W. (1953). Transitional objects and transitional phenomena; A study of the first not-me possession. *International Journal of Psycho-Analysis, 34*, 89–97.

Winnicott, D. W. (1963). Communicating and not communicating leading to a study of certain opposites. In *The maturational processes and the facilitating environment*. New York: International Universities Press, 1965.

Winnicott, D. W. (1965). Ego distortion in terms of true and false self. In *The Maturational Process and the Facilitating Environment: Studies in the Theory of Emotional Development*. New York: International UP Inc.

Winnicott, D. W. (1971a). *Playing and reality*. London: Routledge.

Winnicott, D. W. (1971b). *Therapeutic consultation in child psychiatry*. London: The Hogarth Press and the Institute of Psychoanalysis.

Winnicott, D. W. (1989). *Psycho-analytic explorations*. London: Karnac Books.

Wise, E. H., & Barnett, J. E. (2016). Self-care for psychologists. In J. C. Norcross, G. R. VandenBos & D. K. Freedheim, (Eds.), *APA handbook of clinical psychology: Vol. 5. Education and profession*. Washington, DC: American Psychological Association.

Wittgenstein, L. (1953). *Philosophical investigations.* London: MacMillan.

Yadlin-Gadot, S. (2019). Post-Truth, Hegemonic Discourse and the Psychoanalytic Task of Decentering. Psychoanalytic Dialogues, 29, 172–188.

Yeomans, F.E., Clarkin, J. F., & Kernberg, O. F. (2014). *Transference-focused psychotherapy for borderline personality disorder: A clinical guide.* Washington, DC: American Psychiatric Association.

Yerushalmi, H. (2018). On patients' unique self-knowledge. *International Forum of Psychoanalysis, 27,* 229–240.

Young, J. E., Klosko, J. S., & Weishaar, M. E. (2003). *Schema Therapy: A Practitioner's Guide.* New York: Guilford.

Zetzel, E. R. (1956). Current concepts of transference. *International Journal of Psychoanalysis, 37,* 369–375.

Zilcha-Mano, S. (2019). Major developments in methods addressing for whom may psychotherapy work and why. *Psychotherapy Research, 29(6),* 693–708.

Zilcha-Mano, S. (2021). Toward personalized psychotherapy: the importance of the trait-like/state-like distinction for understanding therapeutic change. *American Psychologist, 76,* 516–528.

Index

For Product Safety Concerns and Information please contact our EU
representative GPSR@taylorandfrancis.com
Taylor & Francis Verlag GmbH, Kaufingerstraße 24, 80331 München, Germany